A Handbook on
Practical Approach to

PANCHAKARMA

(Poorvakarma)

A Handbook on Practical Approach to PANCHAKARMA (Poorvakarma)

SECOND EDITION

Anup Jain MD (Panchakarma)
Assistant Professor
Postgraduate Department of Panchakarma
Chaudhary Brahm Prakash Ayurved Charak Sansthan
New Delhi, India

Foreword

Acharya Tarachand Sharma

JAYPEE The Health Sciences Publisher
New Delhi | London | Panama

JAYPEE **Jaypee Brothers Medical Publishers (P) Ltd.**

Headquarters
Jaypee Brothers Medical Publishers (P) Ltd.
4838/24, Ansari Road, Daryaganj
New Delhi 110 002, India
Phone: +91-11-43574357
Fax: +91-11-43574314
E-mail: jaypee@jaypeebrothers.com

Overseas Offices
J.P. Medical Ltd.
83, Victoria Street, London
SW1H 0HW (UK)
Phone: +44 20 3170 8910
Fax: +44(0) 20 3008 6180
E-mail: info@jpmedpub.com

Jaypee Highlights Medical Publishers Inc.
City of Knowledge, Building 235, 2nd Floor
Clayton, Panama City, Panama
Phone: +1 507-301-0496
Fax: +1 507-301-0499
E-mail: cservice@jphmedical.com

Jaypee Brothers Medical Publishers (P) Ltd.
17/1-B, Babar Road, Block-B, Shaymali
Mohammadpur, Dhaka-1207
Bangladesh
Mobile: +08801912003485
E-mail: jaypeedhaka@gmail.com

Jaypee Brothers Medical Publishers (P) Ltd.
Bhotahity, Kathmandu, Nepal
Phone: +977-9741283608
E-mail: kathmandu@jaypeebrothers.com

Website: www.jaypeebrothers.com
Website: www.jaypeedigital.com

A Handbook on Practical Approach to Panchakarma (Poorvakarma)

Second Edition: **2018**

ISBN: 978-93-5270-253-4

Printed at Replika Press Pvt. Ltd.

Dedicated to

Renowned Nadi Vaidya
Ayurved Dhanvantari of the present era
A source of inspiration to the physicians and faculty of Ayurveda

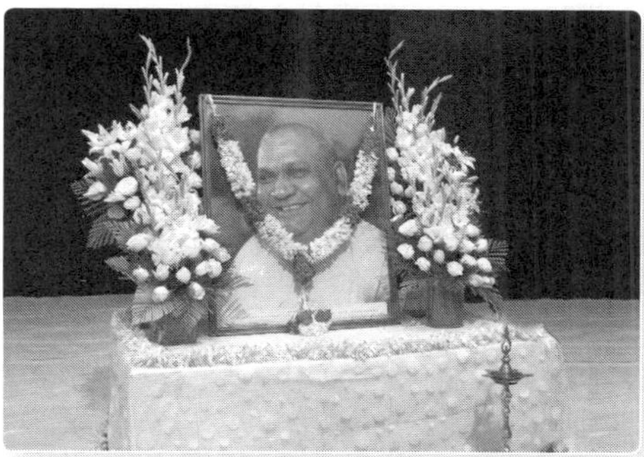

Ayurveda Maharishi, Padma Bhushan and Padma Vibhushan
Late Vaidya Brihaspati Dev Triguna ji

Foreword

There are many *Panchakarma*-related texts published by various *Vaidyas*, but still there is a need for the books which are dedicated to practical aspects of performing *Panchakarma* procedures. These kinds of books can only be written by those who are performing the *Panchakarma* procedures on a regular basis.

The author of *"A Handbook on Practical Approach to Panchakarma (Poorvakarma)"*, Dr Anup Jain, holds a postgraduate degree in *Panchakarma* and working as an Assistant Professor in Postgraduate Department of Panchakarma at Chaudhary Brahm Prakash Ayurved Charak Sansthan, New Delhi, India. The present book is an effort to put his practical experiences and traditional knowledge together. This increases the suitability and value of the book. In this book, the focus has been kept on *Poorvakarma*; types and execution of various procedures under *Snehana* and *Svedana* along with the photographs of the demonstration of his patients. Keeping all these in mind, the book will help the students of *Ayurveda,* who aspire to be *Panchakarma* physicians, general physicians and technicians, who perform the *Panchakarma* procedures in evolving their skills.

I congratulate and wish for the success for the efforts of the author and hope that he will be working on *pradahana karma* and *pashchata karma* as well in the coming times.

Acharya Tarachand Sharma
Ayurvedacharya, MD (Ayurved)
Head
Department of Ayurveda
Model Eye Hospital
Lajpat Nagar, New Delhi, India

Preface

Panchakarma is a branch of *Ayurveda* which for long has been giving tremendous results in clinics and hospitals across the globe. Yet, it has been seen as a complicated science as there are not many texts available, which keep up-to-date, and make it easy for a user to understand, what is required to perform these procedures with clinical precision. There are many texts and details available about the classical approach to *Panchakarma. A Handbook on Practical Approach to Panchakarma (Poorvakarma)* is an effort in the direction to help physicians and train students, who practice *Panchakarma* on practical aspects of performing these procedures with perfection.

This book is dedicated in dealing with the aspect, which is most frequently used in today's era, i.e. the importance of *snehana* and *svedana*. They once have widely been referred to as *Poorvakarma* only; there are many diseases in which they are treatment of choice, i.e. they become *pradhana karma*. The book is also an effort to throw light on the medicines and materials used to give the treatments and also about the kind of diet and regimen which a patient needs to follow, while undergoing the *Panchakarma* therapies.

In the end, I would like to ask for the suggestions and corrections in the book from all the students and Ayurvedic physicians. I assure you that all the suggestions will be studied and corrections incorporated, as education is a lifelong process.

Anup Jain

Acknowledgments

First and foremost, I am thankful to *Lord Dhanvantri,* who imparted the knowledge of *Ayurveda* on earth and without whose blessings none of us would have been having the knowledge of this beautiful science. This book was started with continuous inspiration from great ayurvedic physician Vaidya Acharya Shri Tarachand Sharmaji, my Guru who has taught me over the years in the science of *Ayurveda,* and also who keeps on inspiring me about writing the knowledge we gain, while we study and practice. This book would not have been possible without the blessings of my mentor and great ayurvedic scholar, physician and my Guru Vaidya Shri Rasik S Pawaskar Ji, who nurtured and helped me to understand the theoretical and the practical aspects of clinical approach in *Ayurveda*.

I would also like to thank my parents Smt Sharda and Shri RK Jain, my wife, Dr Namita Jain, and children for their unconditional love and bearing with the time, it takes to write a book and supporting me in every walk of life. I am also thankful to my friends for their support and advice, which helped me to learn and improve the standard of the book. I am also thankful to the management of Chaudhary Brahm Prakash Ayurved Charak Sansthan, especially our Director-Principal Shri Sanjay Giharji, who gave his full support and permissions necessary for compilation and completion of the book.

My sincere gratitude to Shri Jitendar P Vij (Group Chairman), Mr Ankit Vij (Group President), Ms Ritu Sharma (Director-Content Strategy), Ms Sunita Katla (PA to Group Chairman and Publishing Manager), Dr Pinki Chauhan (Development Editor), Ms Seema Dogra (Cover Visualizer), Mr Manoj Pahuja (Graphic Designer), Mohd Iqbal (Typesetter), Mr Ashwani Kumar (Proofreader) and other staff of M/s Jaypee Brothers Medical Publishers (P) Ltd, New Delhi, India, for their support, encouragement and cooperation.

Contents

Plate 1

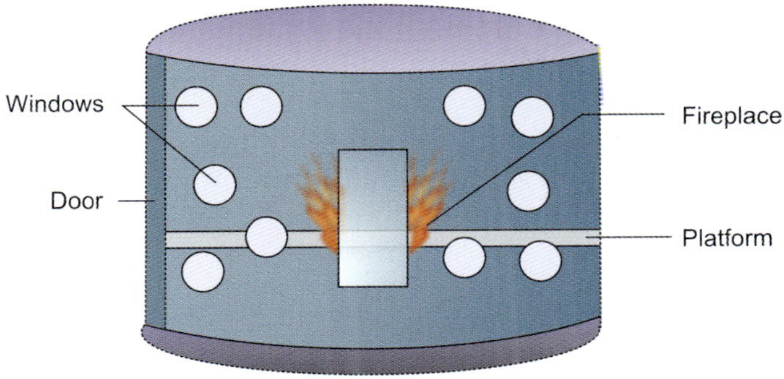

Figure 3.9: *Jentaka sveda kutagara*

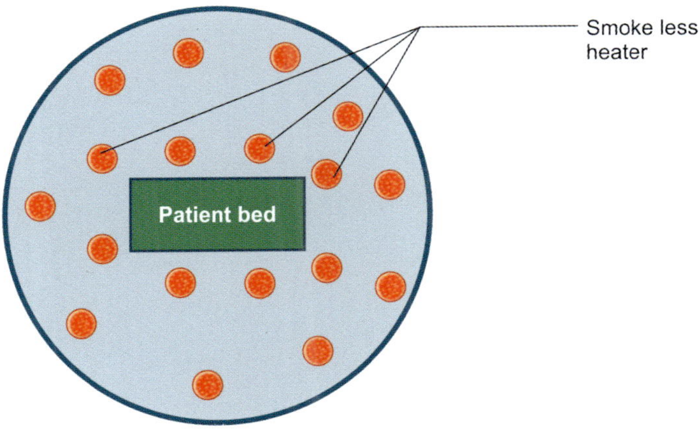

Figure 3.10: *Kuti sveda* (Top view)

CHAPTER

1 Introduction

Panchakarma is a specialised branch of *Ayurveda*, which deals with purification as well as pacification of the *tridosha*, viz. *Vata, Pitta and Kapha* and brings the body to a state of (*Samadosha*) normal health. It is effective in physical as well as mental disorders. *Panchakarma* is not just limited to only *Kayachikitsa* but through its various procedures and ability to cure all types of diseases, this branch has proven that it can help in all the *eight branches* of *Ashtanga Ayurveda*.

The word *panchakarma* is made up from two separate words, i.e. *"Pancha"* and *"Karma"* – '*Pancha*' meaning 'Five' and '*Karma*' meaning work done or treatment procedures. So, *panchakarma* in essentiality means five purification procedures, namely, *Vamana, Virechana, Vasti, Nasya and Raktamokshana*. The word *panchakarma* is mostly used by *Acharya Charaka*; other *Acharyas* like *Vagbhata* and *Sushruta* have not put much emphasis on the word *panchakarma*, although the commentators on these texts have used the term to elaborate the concepts.

SIGNIFICANCE OF PANCHAKARMA THERAPY

Panchakarma is a sort of bio-purification process, also known as *shodhana* therapy in *Ayurveda*, by the administration of which an attempt is made to purify or cleanse all the body tissues (*sroto-shodhana*) and to bring about harmony of *Tridosha*. In broader aspect, we can say it as a body detoxification procedure or technique which cleans the body at the very cellular level.

WHAT IS THE NEED OF PANCHAKARMA?

When the *doshas* are vitiated in such abundance that the palliative treatment is of no help, it is indicated to get rid of excess of vitiated *dosha* by therapeutically eliminating them out of the body.

But these are not the only procedures which this branch is all about. *Panchakarma* is done in three stages—*Poorvakarma, Pradhanakarma* and *Pashchatkarma*. There are plenty of other procedures which are included under the *Poorvakarma* heading of *Panchakarma*. Many of which are independent treatment modalities. In this book, we will try to give the details of all the procedures which come under the heading of *Panchakarma*, their methodology, utility and indications.

Poorvakarma

Poorvakarma includes—Deepana, Pachana, Snehana and *Svedana*.

Deepana and Pachana medicine is given to digest the *Ama dosha* present in the body of a patient and to improve the digestive power (*jatharagni*). It is achieved by giving medicines which improve the digestive power and is done with the help of different medicines. Some of the important medicines which are used for *pachana karma* are *hingwashtaka churna, lavanabhaskara churna, chitrakadi vati, shankha vati, vyoshadi vati* and *lashunadi vati*. Depending upon the requirement as per the digestive power of the patient, *pachana* can be given for 3–5 or more days, depending upon the state of *Ama dosha* and *Jatharagni*.

Signs and Symptoms of Samyak Deepana—Pachana

- *Laghuta* (feeling of lightness in the body)
- *Kshudha Pravritti* (improved appetite)
- *Pipasa* (improved thirst)
- *Nirama Mala Pravritti* (stool without *Ama dosha*)

Snehana is again of two types *Bahya*, i.e. external and *Abhyantara*, i.e. internal. Out of these; internal *snehapana* again can be broadly classified into *vicharana sneha* and *acchapeya sneha*.

Svedana mainly is of two types—*Sagni* and *Niragni*. *Niragni* includes *vayayam*—exercise, *ushna sadan*—sitting in hot room, *guru pravaran*—covering one with heavy woollen clothes, *kshudha*—staying hungry, *bahupan*—drinking hot liquids in excess, *Bhaya*—fear, *Krodha*—anger, *Upanah*—poultice, *Aahav*—wrestling and *Aatap*—sunbath.

Sagni is mainly of four types—*Taapa, upanaha, ushma* and *drava sveda*, which again have many subtypes.

Pradhana Karma

Pradhana karma includes five purification procedures, viz.

1. *Vamana karma (Therapeutic emesis)*: Elimination of vitiated *doshas* through oral route by inducing vomiting is called as *vamana*.

It is very useful in eliminating the excessive *kapha* and is mainly indicated in *kapha dosha pradhana* diseases.

2. *Virechana karma (Therapeutic purgation)*: Elimination of vitiated *doshas* through the anal route by inducing purgation is called as *virechana*. It is very useful in eliminating the excessive *pitta* and is mainly indicated in *pitta dosha pradhana* diseases.
3. *Vasti karma (Medicated enema therapy)*: Administration of medicine through anal, vaginal or urethral route is called *vasti*. It is a very important treatment as it mainly works on *vata dosha*.
4. *Nasya/Shirovirechana karma (Errhine therapy)*: Nasal administration of medicines is called *Nasya*. It is useful mainly in *urdhvajatrugata* diseases.
5. *Raktamokshana karma (Bloodletting therapy)*: Elimination of vitiated *rakta* from the body is called *raktamokshana*. It can be done in six different ways.

Pashchat Karma

Pashchat karma includes Sansarjana krama, Rasayana chikitsa and *Shamana chikitsa* (pacification therapy).

Patients not Suitable for *Panchakarma*

The texts give details of all the indications and contraindications but suggest a few things to keep in mind before we begin a treatment, which is about the patients to reject even if they are indicated for *Panchakarma* treatment. They are:

i. *Anapvad pratikari*: One who keeps arguing and does not follow what his doctor advises.
ii. *Adhana*: Very poor people who cannot afford the medicines.
iii. *Aparicharakavan*: Those who do not have an attendant to take care of them.
iv. *Vaidyamani*: One who thinks of himself as a doctor.
v. *Chanda*: One who does not rest and does stressful and heavy works.
vi. *Asuyaka*: Who is jealous of others.
vii. *Tivradharma aruchi*: Those who are strictly against *panchakarma* or religions.
viii. *Atikshina*: Those who are very weak as they will not be able to bear the harshness of procedures.
ix. *Asadhya roga*: Those with diseases which are described as incurable.
x. *Mumurshalinganvita*: Those who have signs which indicate close end of life.

Acharya Charaka has told the above 10 kinds of people to be rejected for *Panchakarma chikitsa*.

Ashtou Mahadoshakara Vishaya

After this, the texts have also advised to take precautions during the treatment time as well as after a few days, according to the number of days of treatment given, called as *Parihar kala*. They are known as "*Ashtou Mahadoshakara Vishaya*"

These precautions are:
- Do not speak in loud voice.
- Do not travel by horse, elephant or motorbike, scooter, etc.
- Do not travel or walk in excess.
- Do not sit in one position and on one seat for long hours or duration.
- Do not eat before first meal is already digested.
- Do not eat unhealthy and nonsuitable food.
- Do not sleep in day time.
- Do not engage in coitus.

Panchakarma chikitsa is majorly based on *dvividha* or *shadavidha upkrama*. It is important to understand the details of preparation and execution of all the procedures and do them with own hands to achieve proficiency in this subject. In the coming chapters, we will try to summarize the same things.

How to Establish a *Panchakarma* Theatre/Clinic/Hospital?

Detoxification procedure is the main intention and integral part of *panchakarma*. Hence, for the successful achievement of treatment, there must be appropriate equipment and facilities available. May be that is the reason why *Acharya Charaka* has described in his *upakalpaniya adhyaya* that there should be individual rooms/divisions for specific procedure and specific rooms for its collection of drugs and required equipment, so that it is easily accessible when needed. It is also specified to collect the things required, which are necessary for undertaken procedure. By observing this sensitive explanation, proper designing of a hospital/*panchakarma* treatment centre should be done.

Basic Requirements of a Panchakarma Theatre

- The therapy room should be in silent place-void of noise and pollution.
- There must be windows and balcony for proper ventilation.
- Room must be spacious and big enough so that patients/therapists can easily walk around.

- Hospital/clinic should not face to hill or mountain. It should be in such place where there is no direct entry for smoke, sun's harsh rays, water and any kind of dirt.
- There should be sufficient water availability in hospital.
- All necessary equipment should be available.

Apart from this, following divisions and rooms are required to establish a proper *panchakarma* treatment clinic/hospital:

- *Reception cum waiting area*: This area will cater to general inquiries as well as serve as waiting area for outpatient department (OPD) and therapy section of the treatment centre.
- *Equipment and dispensing room*: For *panchakarma* treatment purposes, there should be a room/section where all things are kept systematically, so that they are easily accessible when required. Equipment required are detailed under separate section.
- Therapy Rooms:
  - *For Poorvakarma-Minimum two*: One each for different gender and can be extended in multiples of two or as per the requirement/area available of size 12′ × 12′. They are utilized for simple procedures like *abhyanga, pinda sveda, shirodhara,* etc.
  - *For pradhana karma*: Two/Four rooms with attached toilets—for *vamana, virechana, vasti, nasya* and *raktamokshana*. However, in case of space constraints, a big room can be properly equipped to cater to the different needs of each therapy.
- *Doctor's room*: One for OPD section and one for therapy section.
- *Kitchen*: One for proper preparation of different decoctions and others medicinal requirements of different therapies as discussed in separate chapters.

Equipment(s) Required

- *Therapy tables*: There are different types of therapy tables available for different needs of a treatment centre which are named as:
  - *Abhyanga table* ***(Fig. 1.1)***: It can serve to treatments such as *abhyanga, pinda sveda, sthanik vasti,* etc. where no recollection of oils is required.
  - *Shirodhara table* ***(Fig. 1.2)***: Name of this table explains its uses. Used for various types of *shirodhara* and allied procedures in which recollection of oils/medicines is done only from one end of the table along with the procedures which can be performed on *abhyanga* table.
  - *Droni* ***(Fig. 1.3)***: While supporting all the functions of the first two tables, it also supports pizzichil and similar treatments in which recollection from both ends of the table is required.

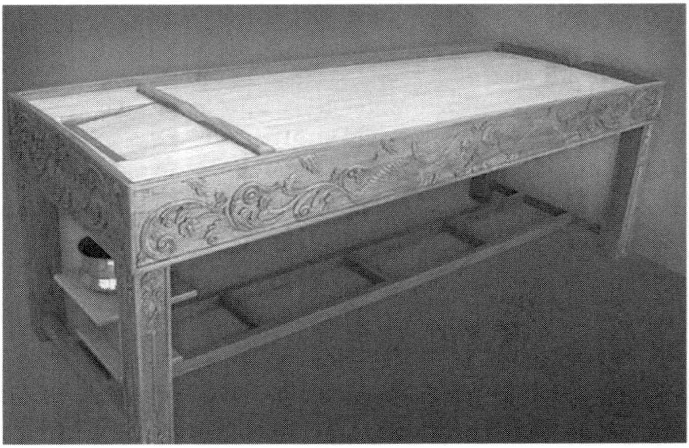

Figure 1.1: *Abhyanga* table

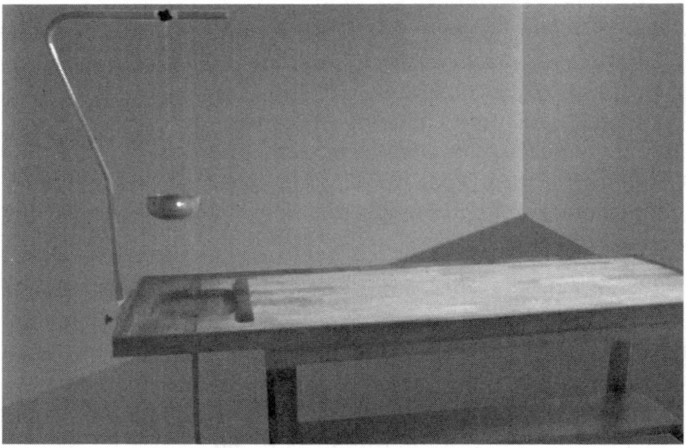

Figure 1.2: *Shirodhara* table

- *Multipurpose table* ***(Figs 1.4 and 1.5)***: Some of the states have developed designs in which many types of treatments can be performed like *bhaya snehana* procedures along with *shirodhara* and *vashpa sveda*.

Note: Requirement of the number of tables in a treatment centre will vary according to the number of rooms available for each section.

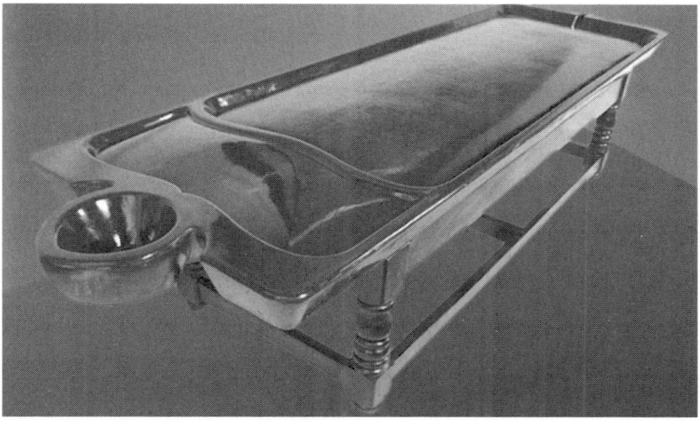

Figure 1.3: *Droni*

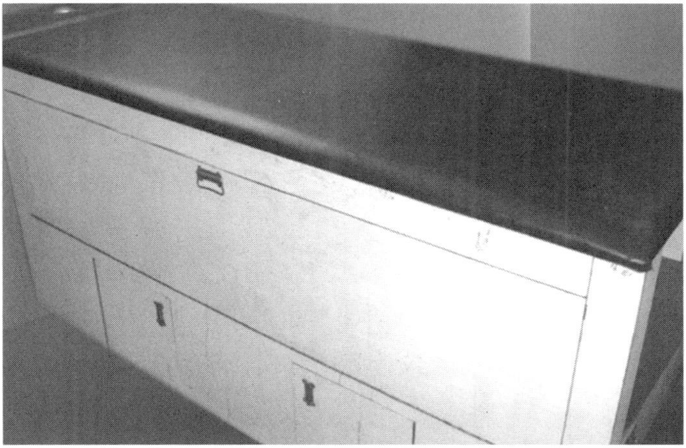

Figure 1.4: Multipurpose table—closed view

- *Sarvanga vashpa svedana yantra (whole body steam chamber/ box)*: To give whole body steam. These are of two types—sitting type **(Fig. 1.6)** and laying down type **(Fig. 1.7)** can be chosen according to the need of the patient.
- *Nadi svedana yantra* ***(Fig. 1.8)***: To give localized steam.

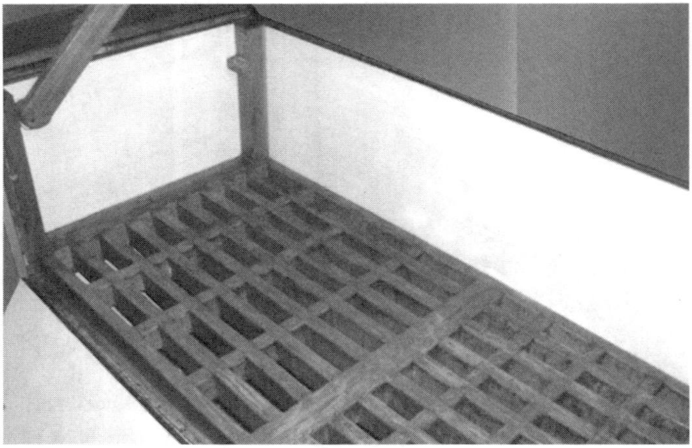

Figure 1.5: Multipurpose table—open

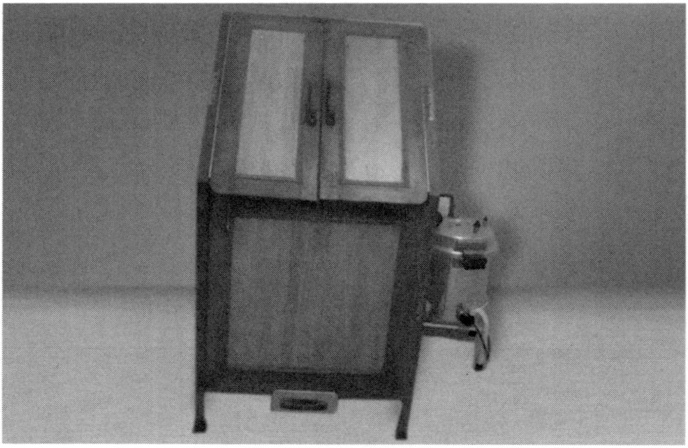

Figure 1.6: *Svedana yantra*—sitting type

- *Steam generators*: Cookers for steam preparation—electric steam generators can be used to serve the purpose of *vashpa svedana*. Alternatively aluminum cookers of size 5 L and above may be used to generate steam.
- *Shirodhara stands* are of three types—table mounted **(Fig. 1.9)**, wall mounted **(Fig. 1.10)** and independent stands **(Fig. 1.11)**. The number and type can be decided according to the space and infrastructure.

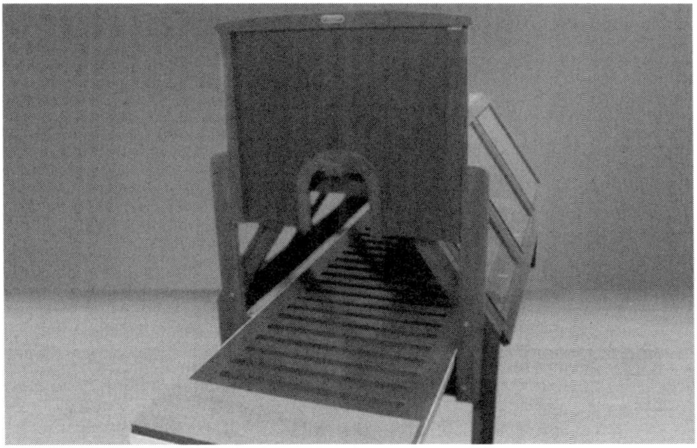

Figure 1.7: *Svedana yantra*—laying down type

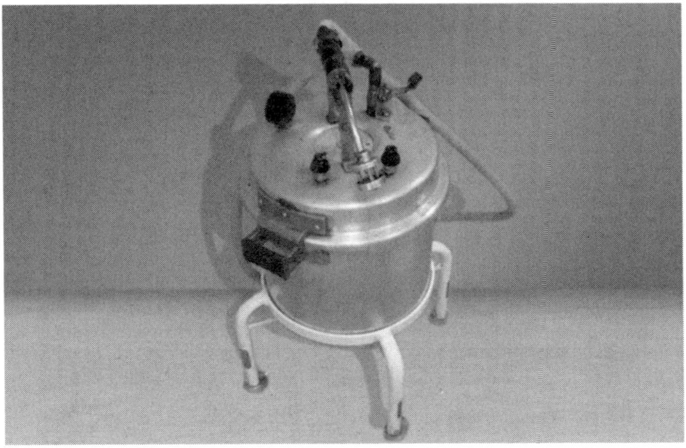

Figure 1.8: *Nadi svedana yantra*

- *Vamana chair/peeth* **(*Fig. 1.12*)**: A knee-high chair with provision of equipment to collect the material of vomitus should be available in *vamana* room.
- *Virechana (Purgation) chair*: It can be placed in toilets or European seats can be used in their absence.

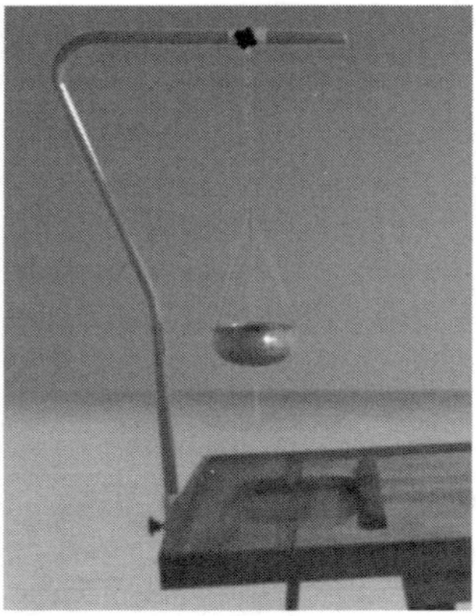

Figure 1.9: *Shirodhara* stand—table mounted

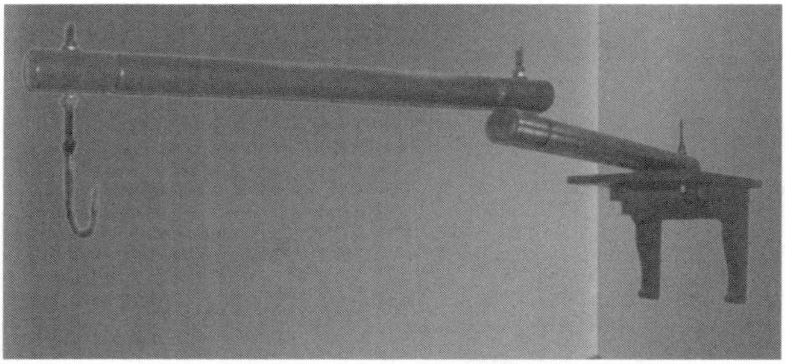

Figure 1.10: *Shirodhara* stand—wall mounted

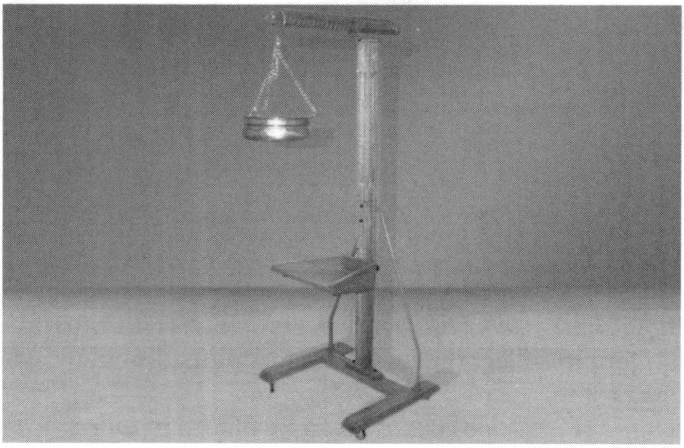

Figure 1.11: *Shirodhara* stand—independent unit

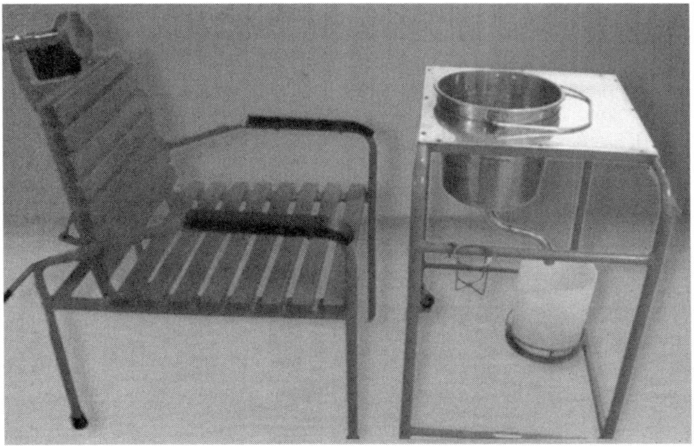

Figure 1.12: *Vamana peeth*

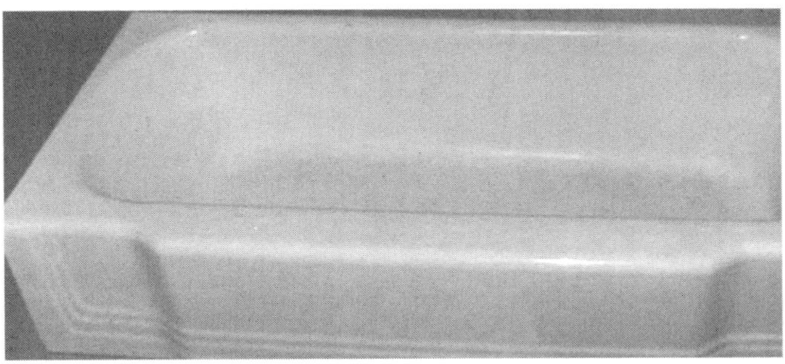

Figure 1.13: *Avagaha yantra*

- *Vasti yantra (Enema equipment/enema can/syringes)*: At least 4 sets with simple rubber catheters in sufficient quantity.
- *Avagaha sveda yantra* ***(Fig. 1.13)***: Tub bath—one for the purpose of *avagahana.*
- *Shirovasti cap* ***(Fig. 1.14)***: One with a knee high armed chair and stepping stool should be available to perform shirovasti.
- *Shirodhara yantra/patra* ***(Figs 1.15A and B)***: These are made of different designs and metals. Should be arranged according to the number of tables supporting *shirodhara.*

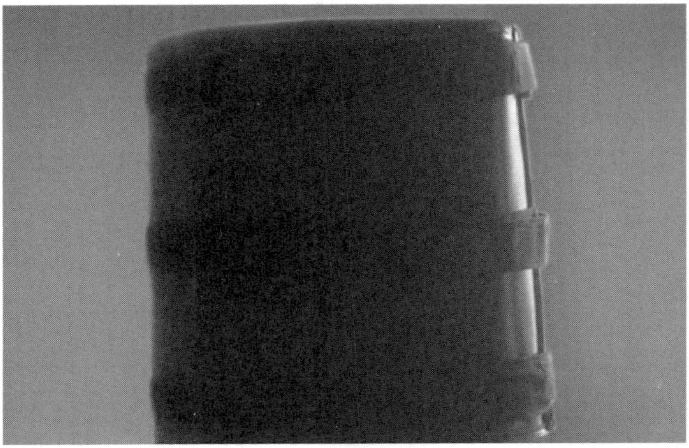

Figure 1.14: *Shirovasti* cap

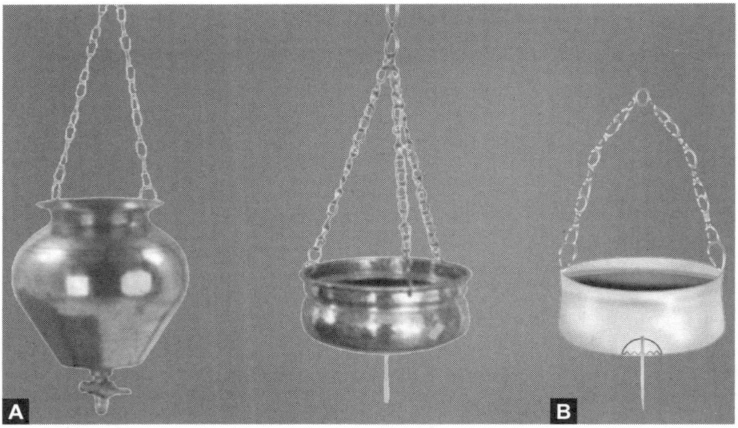

Figures 1.15A and B: *Shirodhara yantra*

- *Nasya peeth:* One—it helps in providing proper position to the patients when administering *nasya*. However, with proper positioning, *abhyanga* table too can be used to administer nasya.
- Other equipment like storage containers, aprons, disposable gloves, gas stoves, heatres, hot plates, bowls and spoons, etc. should be available in sufficient numbers.
- For *raktamokashana*—kidney tray, syringes, cotton and gauge pieces, etc. should be stored in sufficient quantities.

CHAPTER

2 Snehana

Snehana or Oleation therapy means providing lubrication to the body. It is a treatment which brings viscosity, softness, solubility and *kleda* in body. It is essentially of two types as discussed earlier, i.e. internal and external.

Snehana is one of the *Shadvidha upakrama*. Properties of *Snehana dravya* are *snigdha, guru, shita, mridu, drava, picchila, manda* and *Sukshma*.

DEFINITION

The procedure by which body achieves *snigdhata, vishyandata, mardavata* and *kledana* is known as *Snehana*.

PROPERTIES OF SNEHANA DRAVYA

Snehana dravya are *snigdha, drava, mridu, sukshma, sara, picchila* and guru. *Snehana dravya* helps in *vayu nigrahana* and reduces *srotorodha*. All these properties help *snehana dravya* to work efficiently in the body.

The selection and use of *sneha dravya* is primarily done according to *dosha* predominance and the disease condition. Following are a few examples **(Table 2.1)**.

INDICATIONS

People and conditions which are indicated for *Snehana* include the patients who are to be given purification procedures like *Vamana* or *Virechana*, or those who are to be given *Svedana* (Sudation therapy), those who are alcoholic, those who are habitual or indulge in excess intercourse or exercises, those who have stress, old people, children, weak people, those with very dry and thin body, those with weak *rakta* and *shukra dhatu*, those suffering from *vatavyadhi, timira* and *abhishyanda*.

Table 2.1: Use of *Sneha dravya* according to *dosha*

S. No.	*Dosha*	Indicated *dravya*
1.	*Vata*	• *Murchita tila taila* • *Dashmula taila/Ghrita* • *Triphala ghrita*
2.	*Pitta*	• *Ksheerabala taila* • *Mahatikta/Panchatikta ghrita* • *Shatavari ghrita*
3.	*Kapha*	• *Vyoshadi ghrita* • *Triyushnadi ghrita* • *Guggulutiktam ghrita*

Internal *Snehana*

When oleation therapy is given from oral rout, it is called internal or *abhyantara snehana*. It is started only after administering *deepana-pachana* medicine for 3–5 days. There are four categories of *sneha* which can be used for this procedure, viz. *ghrita, taila, vasa* and *majja*. Internal *snehana* is essentially used to prepare a patient for *shodhana*, however in certain conditions, it can also be used for *shamana chikitsa*.

Administration of Snehana According to Seasons

Ghritapana should be done in *sharada ritu, vasa* and *majjapana* should be done in *vasanta ritu* and during rains *taila pana* shall be given. *Snehapana* shall be done when it is neither too hot nor too cold.

Time of Intake of Sneha

During winters, *snehapana* shall be done when the sky is clear during daytime; in summers, it is ideal to administer *snehapana* during night. In people with *vata pittaja prakriti* and diseases *snehapana* shall be given during nighttime and in *vatakaphaja prakriti* and diseases, *snehapana* shall be done in daytime.

Quantity, Anupana and Duration of Snehana

There are three quantities of *snehapana* as advised by different texts—*Pradhana* (high), which takes 24 hours to be digested, *Madhyama* (medium) which takes 12 hours to be digested, and hrasva (low) which takes 6 hours to be digested.

Best *anupana* for *ghritapana* is lukewarm or warm water, *taila pana* is *yusha* and for *vasa* and *majja*, it is *manda*. But warm water can be used for all types of *sneha* as *anupana*.

Abhyantara snehana can be given from days 3 to 7 days according to type of *koshtha*, e.g. a person with *mridu koshtha* should be given *snehapana* only for 3 days and a patient with *krura koshtha* should be given *snehapana* for 7 days. If it is used for more than seven days, the body gets used to it, i.e. body gets *satmya* to *sneha* and its medical properties are not achieved.

Diet before Snehapana

Before starting *snehapana*, patient shall be shifted to food having *drava, ushna* and *anabhishyandi* properties. Also, it is advisable to avoid *viruddha* and *guru ahara*.

Process to Administer Snehana for Shodhana Chikitsa

The sneha to be selected for administration to the patient depends upon the underlying disease **(Table 2.2)**.

It is suggested that snehapana shall be given early in the morning within 15 to 30 minutes of sunrise and the first day's dose is supposed to be *hrasiyasi*, i.e. lesser than the *hrasva* dose. It comes to around 25 mL to 30 mL. Further doses can be administered according to the time it takes to digest this dose. Patients should be counseled in details to make them aware of the different symptoms like nausea, giddiness, etc. they will be going through while taking higher doses of *snehapana*. Doses can be increased by 30 to 40 mL every day according to a patient's condition and time it takes him/her to digest previous day's *sneha*. Dose can be increased up to 250–300 mL in a day on seventh day.

It is often noted that patients are not able to take the initial doses of *snehapana* easily due to *samata*. It is advisable to give *pachana* treatment before initiating the *snehapana*. It can be achieved by giving *chitrakadi vati* or other such *deepana-pachana* drugs for 2 to 3 days.

Table 2.2: Administration of *Snehana* for *shodhana chikitsa*

S. No.	*Sneha Dravya*	Indication
1.	*Tikta ghrita, Mahatikta ghrita* or *Vasa ghrita*	Skin and blood disorders, etc.
2.	*Kalyanaka ghrita, Brahmi ghrita*	Mental disorders, epilepsy, insanity, etc.
3.	*Mahasneha, Panchatikta ghrita, Guggulu*	Paraplegia, etc.

Another precaution or advice we need to provide the patients while administering *sneha* is that the patient shall keep ready some warm water and other material like lemon or *saindhava*. If there is nausea, then the patient can take the help of these materials to sooth the feelings and finish *snehapana*.

Sneha Prakarsha Kala

The *Acharyas* have classified total duration of *snehana* according to *koshtha* which are *mrudu, madhyam* or *krura* as 3, 5 or 7 days respectively. It is said that if *snehana* (i.e. internal *snehana*) is given to a patient for more than 7 days at a stretch, this *sneha* becomes *satmya* to his/her body and therefore, is not advised. It is called *prakarsha kala* of *sneha*.

Signs and Symptoms of Different Stages of Digestion of Sneha

As the *sneha* is administered, different types of signs and symptoms appear during the course of its digestion. According to these, we can reach the conclusion whether the *sneha* is completely digested or not. They are:

Sneha jiryamana lakshana
Signs and symptoms of administered *sneha* being undigested are headache, giddiness, salivation, increased thirst, uneasiness, burning sensation, weakness without doing any work and unconsciousness, etc.

Sneha jirna lakshana
Signs and symptoms of sneha being digested are pacification of above said signs at first, feeling light, *vatanulomana*, feeling hungry, feeling thirsty, and *udgar shuddhi*, i.e. belching is fresh and does not contain odor of sneha.

Signs and Symptoms which Appear during Snehana

When *snehana* is complete, different types of signs and symptoms appear according to the level of *snehana* reached and further course of action is taken accordingly.

Signs and Symptoms of Properly Snigdha People

Improved digestive power (*Agni dipti*), aversion to fat (*snehodwesha*), loose motions (*asanhta varcha*), lightness in body (*anga laghuta*), smoothness in body (*gatra mardawa*), smoothness in body (*snigdha gatrata*), oleus stools (*snigdha purisha*), oleus skin (*snigdha tvak*), passage of flatus (*vatanulomana*), visual fats in stools (*adhstada snehadarshana*), neurasthenia (*klama*), lethargy (*shaithilya*).

Signs and Symptoms of Improperly/Asnigdha People

Stools are dry, hard and difficult to pass, digestive power is low, *vata pratilomatva*, and body is dry. Here we need to understand that the dryness is not formed because of less quantity of *sneha*, but it was already present in the body and did not get cured because of lack of *sneha* absorbed.

Signs and Symptoms of Excessively Snigdha People

Panduta, i.e. anemia like symptoms, viz. pale face eyes and tongue, heaviness in body, feeling cold, stools containing indigested food, weakness, disliking food, nausea, excessive salivation, secretions from anus and burning sensation in anal region.

Pathya–Apathya

Patient is advised to follow *brahmacharya* and take proper posture only. They should avoid variation in temperature, dust, fumes and travelling in open air. They shall not indulge in *vegavrodha* and shall drink only lukewarm water. Also they shall observe *dharana* of *dharaniya vega*.

Pashchat Karma of Snehapana

Food should not contain excess oil or *ghee*, should not be *abhishyandi*, should be *satmya*, not of many types, and only warm water shall be taken. Cold water shall not be used, stools, urine and sneezing should not be stopped, exercises, speaking loudly, being angry and eating cold and old food should be avoided. These precautions shall be taken for the same number of days as *snehapana* is done. If there are any other treatments planned after *snehana*, i.e. if *snehana* is done as *poorvakarma* they can be planned as per the following guidelines.

Purification and sudation treatments after snehana

When there is *avara snehana*, sudation shall be done on the fourth day, in case of *madhyama snehana*, *svedana* shall be done from fifth day, and in case of *pravara snehana*, *svedana* shall be done from eighth day. When *vamana* is to be given, one day's gap shall be taken after *snehapana* ends. In case of *virechana*, three days gap shall be given. During the gap or rest days proper diet and *svedana* shall be done. When *vasti* is to be done, it is advised that *snehapana* is not required because all the *vastis* contain some form of *sneha* in them, and it is contraindicated to give *sneha* from oral and rectal routes together.

External *Snehana*

When oleation therapy is given from external route it is called as external or *bhaya snehana*. Many of these procedures can be used independently as a treatment module in many diseases. This kind of *snehana* is very useful as *pradhana karma,* so details are being discussed for each of them one by one. These treatments are more popular in today's time by the term *panchakarma* than the real *shodhana* procedures.

Abhyanga or Tailabhyanga

It means application/massage of oil, etc. over the body. It can be used for not only curing the diseases but also to attain good health and to prevent diseases. It is described as a part of *swasthavritta* in *dincharya* description of all the texts **(Fig. 2.1)**.

Abhyanga acts directly over the largest organ of our body, i.e. skin, which is also *adhishthana* of *vata dosha*. It is said that a person shall do *abhyanga* daily to stay healthy.

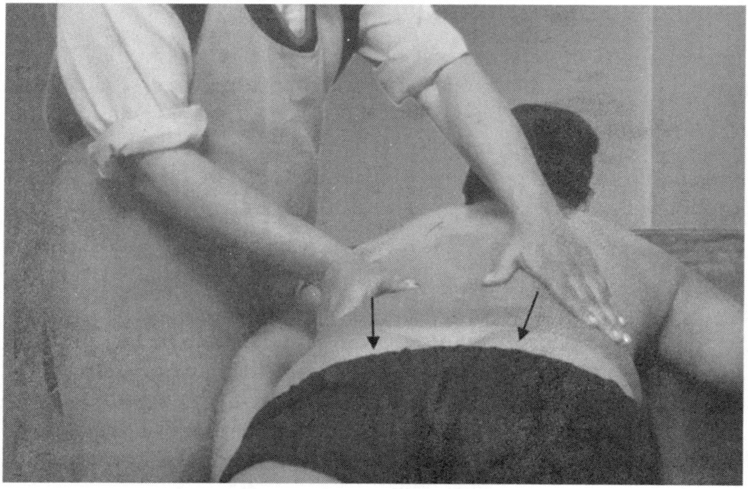

Figure 2.1: *Abhyanga*

Contraindications

As described above, *abhyanga* is included in the daily regimen, so it is indicated to be used on everyone barring a few conditions which we need to keep in mind. They are people suffering from:

- Kaphaja diseases
- Those that have just been given *vamana, virechana* or *vasti*
- Those suffering from indigestion
- Those having *samata* or *sama vyadhi*
- Those having *navajvara*
- Those having *santarpanotha* diseases.
- *Raktapitta*
- *Atisara*

Medicines required

Depending upon the involvement of *dosha*, various types of oils can be used for *abhyanga* therapy as indicated here:

- Oils used for head massage
  - *Chandanadi taila*
  - *Brahmi taila*
  - *Jyotishmati taila*
  - *Nilgiri taila*
  - *Himsagara taila*
- Oils used for body massage
  - *Vataja disorders: Narayana taila, Bala taila, Dashmula taila,* etc.
  - *Pittaja disorders: Kshirabala taila, chandanadi taila, chandanabala-lakshadi taila,* etc.
  - *Kaphaja disorders: Sahacharadi taila, nirgundi taila, Dashmula taila,* etc.

Materials required

Abhyanga table, bowls, heater, napkins, plastic apron.

Preparation

Following method should be adopted for heating oil not only for *abhyanga* but for all the procedures:

- Take heated steel bowl and fill it with an oil, or
- Fill a bowl with oil and then heat the bowl by putting it in hot water.

Procedure

Ashtanga hridaya states that *abhyanga* should be done over head, ears and feet. For massaging head, normal or lukewarm oil should be used. Rest of the body should be massaged with lukewarm oils. In cold, season, *ushna gunatmaka taila;* and in hot seasons *shita gunatmaka taila* should be used.

Tailabhyanga should always be done in *anuloma gati* (i.e. from above—downward direction) especially on body parts such as arms, forearms, thighs, legs, scapular region, upper back, lower back, chest and abdomen, and in *vartulakar* (clockwise circular movements) on joints such as shoulder, elbow, knee, ankle and vertebral column, etc.

Therapist should be aware of the functions of all the body parts and also of every muscle. He should do *abhyanga* in such a manner that it is beneficial to functionality of each and every muscle.

Generally, on *ekanga* (restricted part) *tailabhyanga* should be done for 5–7 minutes. On *sarvanga* (full body) *tailabhyanga* should be done from 30–45 minutes or more if required. After *tailabhyanga,* the patient should be advised to take 15 minutes rest. Clean the oil from body with cotton cloth and only after 1 hour, the patient should take bath with warm/hot water using green gram powder instead of soap. This procedure is continued for 7 days or more.

For doing good tailabhyanga on every part, following 7 postures should be used:

1. **Sitting:** Seated with both legs extended. In this position, first apply oil on head, ears (*Karna purana*), umbilicus, palms and soles. Then *tailabhyanga* of vertebral column, scapular region, upper and lower back and upper extremities should be done **(Figs 2.2 and 2.3)**.
2. **Supine:** Lying on the back side of the body. In this position, *tailabhyanga* of right and left side of chest is done along with abdomen, anterior side of the right and left upper extremity as well as of lower extremities is also done **(Fig. 2.4)**.

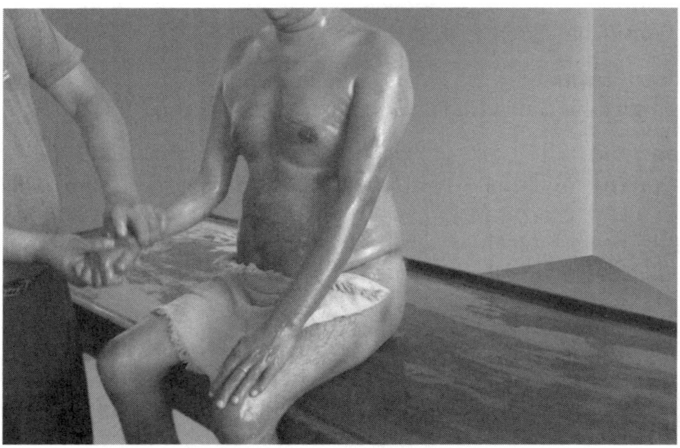

Figure 2.2: Sitting posture 1

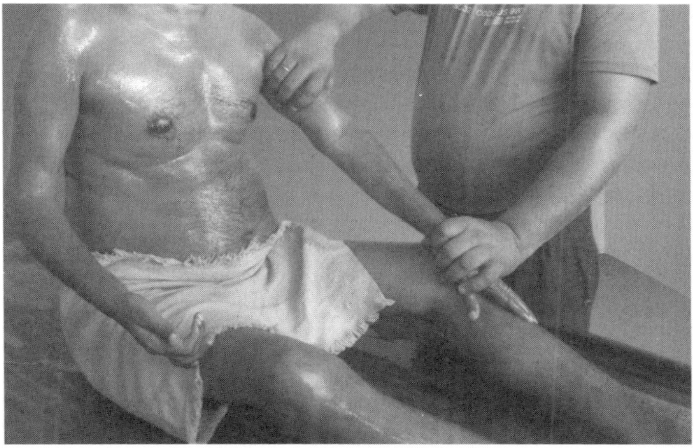

Figure 2.3: Sitting posture 2

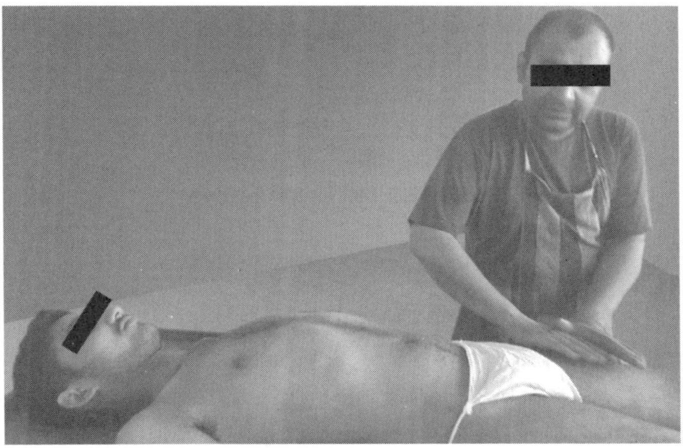

Figure 2.4: Supine posture

3. **Left lateral:** Lying on the left side of the body with left lower extremity extended and right lower extremity is in semiflexion at hip and knee. In this position, *tailabhyanga* is done on right lateral side of chest, abdomen, right lower extremity and medial side of left lower extremity **(Fig. 2.5)**.
4. **Prone:** Lying on the front side of the body. In this position, *tailabhyanga* is done on scapular region, upper and lower back,

lateral sides of chest and abdomen and on posterior sides of the lower extremity **(Fig. 2.6)**.

5. **Right lateral:** Lying on the right side of the body with right lower extremity extended and left lower extremity semiflexed at hip and knee. In this position *tailabhyanga* is done on lateral side of chest and abdomen, left lower extremity and on medial side of right lower extremity **(Fig. 2.7)**.

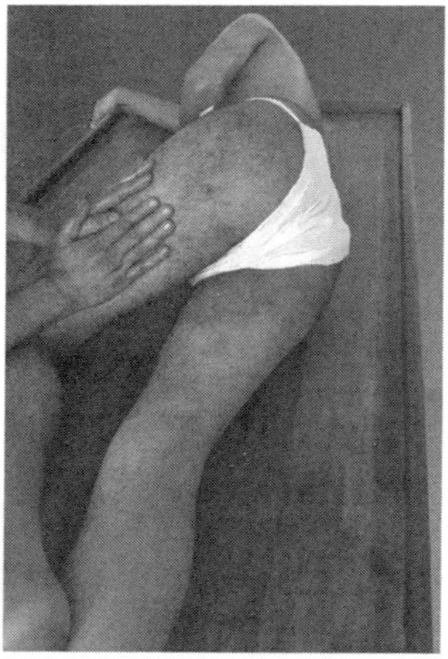

Figure 2.5: Left lateral posture

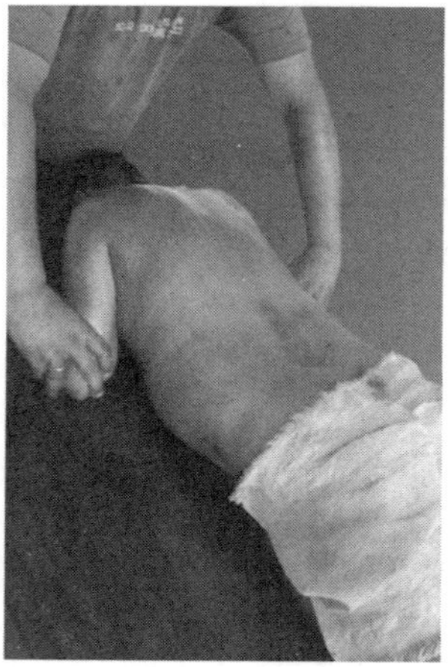

Figure 2.6: Prone posture

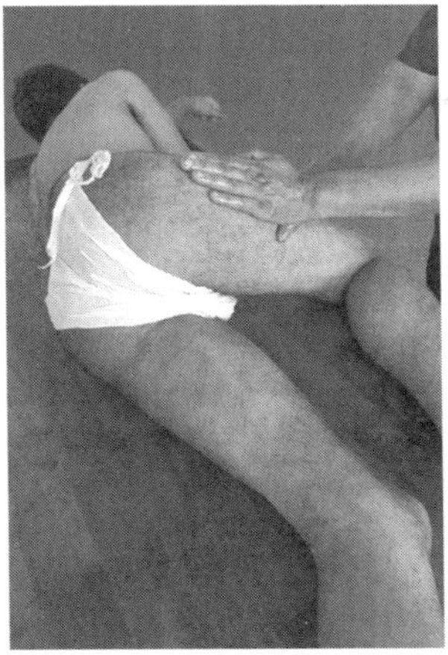

Figure 2.7: Right lateral posture

6. Repeat posture no. 2, i.e. supine
7. Repeat posture no. 1, i.e. sitting.

Uses and properties

- *Abhyanga* reduces aging (by improving strength of *dhatu*) and tiredness.
- *Abhyanga* pacifies *vata dosha*, improves vision, increases life expectancy and induces sound sleep.
- *Tailabhyanga* of the body imparts glossy soft appearance to the skin.
- Protects against vitiation and aggravations of *vata* and *kapha*.
- Improves color and strength of the body.
- Tones up the *dhatu* (basic principles/root principles of the body)
- *Vata dosha* pre-dominates the tactile sensory organs which are lodged in the skin. *Abhyanga* is very useful to skin if practised regularly.
- In diseases like *sandhigata vata, grudhrasi, khalli, katistambha* and *shula, manya stambha* and *shula, khanja, apabahuka, hasta pada shula* and *chimchimayana, abhyanga* proves to be a very good modality.

Thalodala

It is a type of deep tissue massage which is famous in South India. In this treatment, the pressure applied over the body is more than that in *abhyanga* and thus it results in deeper permeation of oils **(Fig. 2.8)**.

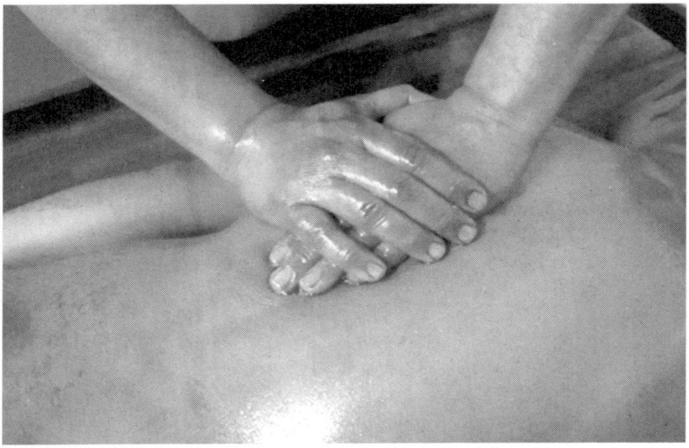

Figure 2.8: Thalodala

Medicines required
Medicated oils.

Materials required
Droni, bowls, heater, napkins, plastic apron.

Preparation
Standard method shall be followed to heat the oil.

Procedure
First oil shall be applied on head, ears, umbilicus, foot, palm and whole body. *Thalodala* should be done with a continuous pressure of about 1 cm from skin surface and is done in following three phases:

Phase one: It has following steps in it:

- Patient is asked to lie down in prone position. In this position, both the hands are at first placed on the lumbar region and moved into and fro movements.
- In next step, hands are moved in upward direction up to the shoulder level, then extending towards the right parallel to spine segment by segment. After completing right side, same procedure is repeated on the left side.
- In next step, the hands move from right to left and from left to right making an arch in between.
- Then the hands are moved diagonally connecting right and left corners.

- After completing back massage, hands are moved making an arch from one popliteal fossa to another.
- In the last step, the arch is extended to cover calcanium.

Phase two: It has following steps in it:

- Patient is asked to lie down in supine position. In this, first massage is done on umbilicus in circular movements.
- In next step, massage is done on chest in circular movements.
- In next step, anterior aspect of both legs is massaged with arch movements from right side to left side.

Phase three: It has following steps in it:

- Patient is asked to sit. In this first massage is done on both the arms separately while being extended laterally.
- In next step, massage is done on neck, head and face. In this position the physician should stand behind the patient and bend the head a little backward.

Important points to remember

- Massage should be a continuous and gentle process.
- Pressure should be applied uniformly throughout the course.
- In every step, process should be repeated at least 3 times.
- Patient shall be rested for at least one hour after the treatment.

Uses

- It helps in reducing the spasm of muscles.
- Reduces painful conditions.
- It is also beneficial in many lower back and spinal diseases.
- It also increases flexibility of body.
- Reduces fatigue and stress.

Udvartana/Utsadana

It means doing *abhyanga* with a specific pressure and in *pratiloma* direction, i.e. from below upwards. It is of two types—*Snigdha* and *Ruksha*. *Ruksha udvartana* is also called as *churnodvartana*. It is indicated in obesity and helps in cleansing the skin and is also a beauty treatment which exfoliates the dead skin and nourishes the healthy skin tissue **(Fig. 2.9)**.

Indications

Ruksha udvartana is done in *Sthaulya chikitsa*, to cleanse the body and to improve the texture of skin. *Snigdha udvartana* is done for underweight people and to achieve *varna prasadan*.

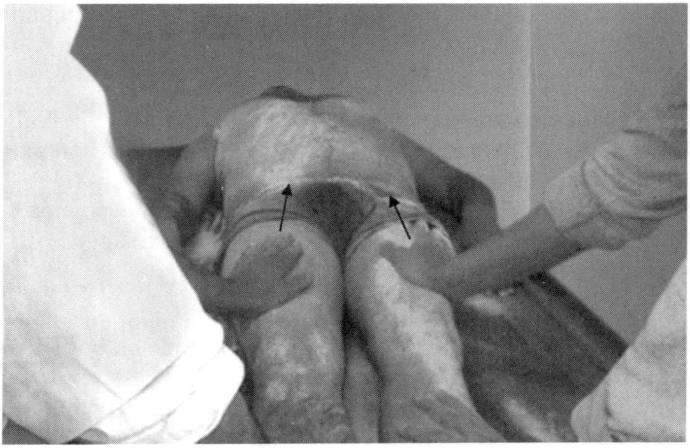

Figure 2.9: Udvartana

Medicines required

- For *snigdha udvartana*: Vatahara oils, e.g. *Dhanwantara* or *bala taila*
- For *ruksha udvartana: Kaphahara churna* like *Kolakulathadi churna, triphala churna, kottamchukkadi churna,* etc.

Materials required

Abhyanga table, bowls, heater, napkins, plastic apron.

Preparation

- *For snigdha udvartana*: Standard method should be adopted for heating oil as described earlier.
- *For ruksha udvartana*: There are two ways to do *ruksha udvartana*:
  - *For people with delicate skin:* Mix the dry powder with some warm *vata kapha nashak* oil, like *triphaladi taila,* etc.
  - *For people with normal skin:* Use the *churna* directly after heating it.

Procedure

Udvartana should always be done in *pratiloma gati* (i.e. from below—upward direction) especially on body parts such as arms, forearms, thighs, legs, scapular region, upper back, lower back, chest and abdomen, and in *vartulakar* (clockwise circular movements) on joints such as shoulder, elbow, knee, ankle and vertebral column, etc. Special care shall be taken while performing *udvartana* on abdomen as important vital organs are situated there and pressure shall be given accordingly. To achieve weight loss, it is important that ideal pressure be applied over abdomen in a way that will help in metabolism of subcutaneous fat. For weight gain, it is important that we give right pressure throughout the body.

Generally, on each part *udvartana* should be done for 3–5 minutes. On *sarvanga* (full body) *tailabhyanga* should be done for about 40 minutes or more if required. After *udvartana*, the patient should be advised to take 15 minutes rest. Clean the oil from body with cotton cloth and only then the patient should take bath with warm/hot water using green gram powder instead of soap. This procedure is continued for 7 days or more.

Uses

- *Udvartana* cleanses all the pores of the body and thus improves health as well as texture and tone of skin (Tvak prasadana).
- *Udvartana* pacifies *kapha, vata* and also melts excessive *meda dhatu*.
- *Udvartana* brings lightness to body and gives weight reduction.
- Reduces the bad odor of the body by cleaning the remnants of sweat and dirt.
- Increases alertness by reducing the *kapha dosha*.
- Reduces itching over body.
- Improves the digestive power present in skin hence, helping in better absorption of lepa, etc. being done to improve the beauty of a person.

Mardana–Unmardana

It is a procedure in which considerable pressure is given while doing massage therapy. In some texts it is written that *mardana* shall be done after doing *abhyanga*. *Mardana* can be done either with or without oils. *Mardana* means pressing the parts downwards and *unmardana* means pulling them upwards. Usually both these treatments are done together to achieve better results. *Mardana* is also done from one end of a muscle to the other to release the spasms.

Indications

It can be done in *vatavyadhi* like *tvakagata vata, mansagata vata, raktagatvata, siragata vata, snayu-sandhi-asthigata vata*, etc. It is also beneficial in spondylitis, muscular spasms and certain painful conditions. It removes the fatigue of muscles and relieves neuralgia.

Medicines required

Vatashamaka or disease specific oils if required.

Materials required

Abhyanga table, bowls, heater, napkins, plastic apron.

Preparation
Standard method should be adopted for heating oil as described earlier.

Procedure
Mardana—*unmardana* are done after massage has been done. After completing *abhyanga, mardana* and *unmardana* are done by pressing into the skin and then lifting a muscle up. It is especially beneficial if *unmardana* is done from one end of a muscle to the other end.

Uses
- It helps in reducing the spasm of muscles
- Reduces painful conditions.
- Helps in curing various types of *vatavyadhi* as cited above.

Padaghata

It is a massage which is done by considerable pressure of feet. A trained masseur is required to complete this treatment as it requires great expertise and balance of the body. It is famous in southern India as *Chaveti*. The person who performs this should not be too thin or too fat, his/her feet shall be soft, smooth and should not be cracked, rough or hard.

Indications
It can be done at the end of day to reduce tiredness, to increase strength of body, as a relaxing and rejuvenating treatment, after exercises, after *abhyanga* in *hemanta ritu* as part of *ritucharya*.

Medicines required
Vatashamaka or disease-specific oils if required.

Materials required
One soft mat for the patient, two rough coconut mats to be placed on either side of the first mat, *abhyanga* table, bowls, heater, napkins, plastic apron, ropes which are tied to the ceiling.

Preparation
Standard method should be adopted for heating oil as described earlier. *Padaghata* is started only after patient has been properly anointed already.

Procedure
At first the body of patient is properly anointed. After that there are two ways to perform *padaghata*, one is on the table and other is on the floor. Mats are required if the procedure is being done on the floor and if the procedure is being performed on the table they are not required. Ropes are tied with the roof and should be long, strong and soft enough for

the therapists to hold without having the risk of hands slipping or the rope breaking. Deep massage is done on back and legs by using toes and complete foot of the therapist without hurting the patient.

Uses

- It helps in reducing the spasm of muscles.
- Reduces painful conditions.
- It increases the strength of the body and prevents diseases.
- It is also beneficial in many lower back and spinal diseases.
- It also increases flexibility of body.
- Reduces fatigue and stress.

Parisheka

In general, it means pouring the stream of a hot or warm liquid, whether a decoction, milk, water, *ghrita, takra* or oil over the body. It is also called as *seka, sechana, parishechana, kayaseka,* etc. It requires higher amounts of *sneha* and can also be considered as a part of *snigdha svedana* as the heat is given by the hot oils which are continuously poured over the body.

Indications

Vatarakta, vatavyadhi, tiredness, *asthibhagna,* blunt injuries, etc.

Medicines required

Vatashamak or disease-specific oils, if required.

Materials required

Abhyanga table, bowls, heater, napkins, plastic apron, cloth piece of 18" × 18" or sponge pieces, *dharapatra.*

Preparation

Standard method should be adopted for heating oil as described earlier.

Procedure

At first, the body of the patient is properly anointed. While doing *parisheka,* proper temperature shall be maintained. The warm oil is gently poured over the affected area or over the whole body as per the requirement. This procedure takes 10–15 minutes for *ekanga* and about 45–60 minutes for *sarvanga parisheka.* After the treatment is done, the patient shall be cleaned properly and be allowed to rest for some time.

Uses

- It helps in curing *vatarakta, vatavyadhi* and *bhagna.*
- Nourishes the body just like water nourishes plants.
- Relieves the pain due to any cause.

Samvahana

Samvahana means soothing and soft touch. It is a light variety of *snehana*. *Samvahana* means light and healing touch. Its procedure is similar to *abhyanga* but for not having the seven postures and also with very low pressure.

Indications
Insomnia, stress and tiredness, etc.

Medicines required
Vatashamak or disease-specific oils, if required.

Materials required
Abhyanga table, bowls, heater, napkins, plastic apron.

Preparation
Standard method should be adopted for heating oil as described earlier.

Procedure
Samvahana is done by doing massage with very light and healing touch. Many texts include it is the *dincharya* regimen. It is done in *anuloma disha* on body and *vartulakar disha* over joints. Care shall be taken to not to apply pressure as it is done by simple caressing technique.

Uses
- It gives light and relaxing feeling and improves the quality of *mansa, rakta* and *tvacha*.
- Induces normal sleep.
- Pacifies *kapha* and *vata*.
- Reduces stress and tiredness.
- It increases affection and nourishes the *dhatus*.

Murdha Taila

Applying oil over head is called *murdha taila*. It is of four types as under:
1. *Shirobhyanga*
2. *Shirahseka*
3. *Shirohpichu*
4. *Shirovasti*

While giving details and properties of *murdha taila,* it is said that applying oil daily over head helps in prevention of headache, delays greying of hair and provides strength to skull and hair. Beautifies the skin of face and induces normal, sound sleep. These four types of treatment are more beneficial than the other in the same order, i.e. *Shirobhyanga, shirahseka, shirohpichu* and *shirovasti*.

1. *Shirobhyanga*

Massaging oil over head is called as *shiro-abhyanga*. It is advisable to use lukewarm or normal temperature oil for this. Normally *abhyanga* is also stated by applying oil over the head first. *Shirah* is said to be *moolasthan* of all the *indriya*. By doing *shirobhyanga* daily, we can achieve the following:

- Long and healthy hair
- Healthy *indriya*
- Beautiful skin of face
- Sound sleep
- It is distressing.

2. *Shirahseka/Shirodhara*

Pouring of warm liquids on head, especially forehead is called as *Shirahseka*. It is also called as *shirodhara*. It is useful in many diseases and can be done with various liquids like decoction, *ghrita*, milk, oil, etc. **(Fig. 2.10)**.

Indications

Headache, stress, insomnia, anxiety and different types of *shiroroga* like *shankhaka, ardhavabhedaka, suryavarta,* etc.

Medicines required

Vatashamak or disease specific oils/decoctions/milk, etc.

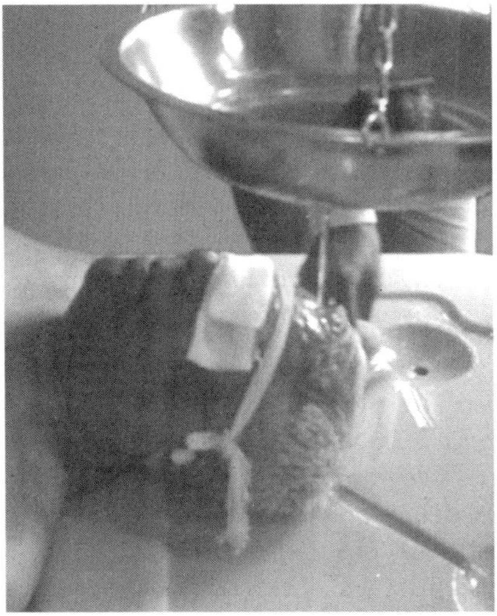

Figure 2.10: *Shirodhara*

Materials required

Shirodhara table, dharapatra, bowls, heater, napkins, plastic apron, cotton.

Preparation

Standard method should be adopted for heating oil as described earlier.

Procedure

A total of 1240 mL of liquid is required to do this treatment. This liquid shall be lukewarm when being used to give *shirodhara. Shirodhara* shall be done only after completing *abhyanga,* etc. procedures if prescribed to the patient. His eyes and ear shall be covered with cotton and if required they can be tied lightly to hold them in place. The liquid shall be filled carefully in the *dharapatra* so as it doesn't get spilled around. After this, there shall be another bowl placed under the head side of *dhara* table, where we can collect the liquid to reuse it.

Shirodhara shall be done in a silent atmosphere in the morning hours before sun reaches its peak. If not in this time, it can be done in the evening when the sun starts setting, but not at night. *Varti* from the *dharapatra* shall be placed at about 4 *angula* from the forehead of the patient. *Dhara* falling over the forehead shall be constant and not very slow or very fast. Also the volume of *dhara* at one time shall not be high. *Dhara* shall be started at the center of the forehead and simple oscillatory movements shall be given to *dharapatra* so that the oils are poured across the forehead stimulating and having effect on all of head. Light and gentle stroking of head can be done, and the recollected liquids shall be warmed again and mixed with the already existing liquids in *dharapatra.*

Different types of medicated liquids which can be used according to different diseases as told by Dharakalpa are—*Tila taila* in *vata* and *kapha dosha, ghrita* in *rakta* and *pitta, Yamaka* of oil and *ghrita* in *vata* and *rakta* and *vata* and *pitta* diseases, also milk can be used in fever—like conditions and *takradhara* in various *vata* and skin diseases. At the end of treatment, head should be dried and *rasna churna* should be applied over *brahmarandhra* to protect *shirastha marma.*

Uses

- It is helpful in curing various *shiroroga* like *ardhavabedaka, shankhaka, suryavarta,* etc.
- Induces normal sleep and reduces stress and anxiety.
- Nourishes hair, delays greying and hairfall.
- Improves memory by nourishing brain.
- Helps in curing various diseases such as *pakshaghata, ardita, nidra nasha,* etc.

- It produces tranquility of mind by calming down the sympathetic activity.
- Rejuvenating effect on brain tissue which is the seat of learning and memory.

There is a special way of doing *shirodhara* with *takra* which requires special citation here so we are describing it in detail. The methodology of *takradhara* is similar to *shirodhara* but the difference is in preparation of medicine.

Takradhara

It is a special type of *shirodhara* which is done by *takra* made in a unique way. It is very popular in Kerala.

Indications
Khalitya, palitya, shirahshula, psoriasis, *hridaroga, aruchi, agnimandya, karnaroga, netraroga.*

Medicines required
Amalaki kvatha and takra

Materials required
Shirodhara table, *dharapatra,* bowls, heater, napkins, plastic apron, cotton.

Preparation
To prepare *amlaki kvatha,* we need about 80 *tola amlaki churna* made of *amlaki* without seeds. Then we add 228 *tola* water to it and boil till 1/4th remains which comes to about 57 *tola*. Preparing *takra* needs a special understanding. Take milk 128 *tola,* and add four times (512 *tola*) water and *musta churna* 8 *tola*. All of these shall be heated till only milk is left which comes to about 128 *tola*. This milk shall then be converted into curd and *takra* made out of it. Freshly prepared *amlaki kvatha* is added to this and our medicine for *takradhara* is ready.

Procedure
It is similar to *shirodhara*.

Uses
- Delays greying of hair and arrests hair fall
- Cures dandruff
- Reduces headache
- It is a very good treatment for diseases such as psoriasis, *hridaroga, agnimandya* and *aruchi*
- It also helps in curing certain *karna roga* and *netraroga*
- Helps in curing insomnia, stress and tiredness.

3. *Shirahpichu (Shiropichu)*

Keeping a cotton or gauge piece soaked in medicated oil or *ghee* is called as *pichudharana*. It is kept over *brahmarandhra* (anterior *fontanelle*). It is helpful is different kinds of *shiroroga*, many scalp-related diseases, dandruff, hair fall, greying of hair, injury to scalp and in many *netra roga*. It is important to keep in mind that *shiropichu* is contraindicated in patients suffering from *peenasa*.

Medicines required

Prescribed *sneha, rasnadi churnam*

Materials required

Cotton, stove, bowls and vessels, towels, gauze

Preparation

Ideally the patient who is advised *shiropichu* should shave his head for better results. Alternatively, this treatment can be done with hair too.

Procedure

To begin with, light head massage is done on the patient with lukewarm oil. A cotton pad which is soaked in the prescribed oil is placed over the head of the patient at *brahmrandhra* region and tied with the help of gauze piece while taking care that the oil should not pour out. This *pichu* is kept for about 30 minutes and can be applied for the required number of days.

Uses

It is useful in patients suffering from various types of shiroroga especially *vataja shiroroga*, hair loss, premature greying of hair, *daha, manyastambha, dandaa-ptanaka* and other psychological diseases.

4. *Shirovasti*

It is the fourth type of *murdha taila*. In this, leather caps open on the top are used to keep the oil filled over the head **(Figs 2.11 and 2.12).**

Indications

Loss of sensation in head or body, *ardita, karnaroga, netraroga, anidra,* and *ardhavabhedaka,* etc.

Medicines required

Medicated oil as per requirement

Materials required

A chair of proper height, *shirovasti* cap, bandage, black gram flour, cotton, bowl, heater and spoons

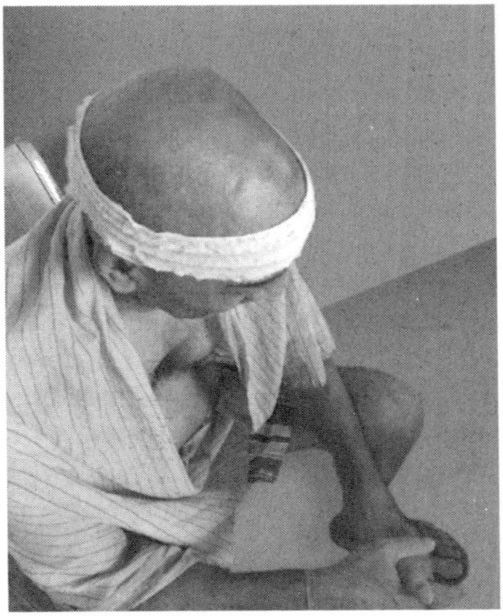

Figure 2.11: *Patta bandhan* before *Shirovasti*

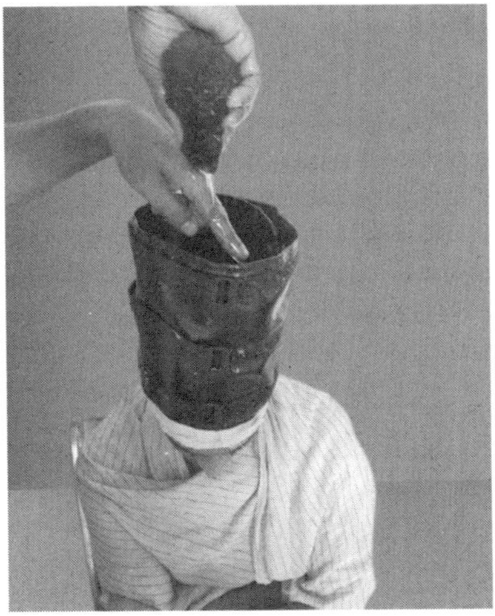

Figure 2.12: Applying *Shirovasti*

Preparation

The head of the patient should be shaved before *shirovasti* if possible as it helps in better procedure execution and also in better absorption of the medicated oils. After that, the patient is given *abhyanga svedana* as per requirement.

Procedure

While applying *shirovasti*, the patient shall be seated on a *janutulyasana* so that his posture is stable and he will not get unbalanced while the treatment is being done. *Shirovasti* cap is of about 12 *angula* height and with diameter similar to head. It is placed and tied over forehead. Black gram flour is used to fill up the gaps and fix it properly so that the filled oils will not leak out of it. Similarly, paste of black gram flour is applied from outside also so that there are no chances of oil leaking out of the cap. Patient should be informed to not to move or tilt his head while the treatment is underway. Lukewarm oil should be filled to the height of two fingers above scalp. Oil shall be taken out and refilled with warm oil so that the temperature is maintained throughout the procedure. When duration of *shirovasti* is complete, all of the oil shall be removed and then *samvahana* of shoulders, neck and head should be done.

Duration of shirovasti according to diseases

- *Vata pradhana* diseases - 10000 *matra* which is about 53 minutes
- *Pitta pradhana* diseases - 8000 *matra* which is about 43 minutes
- *Kapha pradhana* diseases - 6000 *matra* which is about 31 minutes

Uses

- *Shirovasti* is the best type of *murdha taila*
- Gives good results in all types of *shiroroga*
- Reduces stress, anxiety and insomnia
- Improves circulation in head and perception of sense organs
- Is useful in *nasashosha, asyashosha, timira, daruna,* etc.
- It also helps in curing facial paralysis.

Akshi Tarpana

The procedure in which *sneha* is filled over eyes is called as *akshi tarpana* **(Fig. 2.13)**.

Indications

Timira, netrastabdhata, netrarukshta, netrabhigata, netra jimhata (squint), *krichronmilan* (difficulty in opening and closing eyelids), *avilekshana* (blurred vision), *abhishyanda, adhimantha, arjuna—netra roga, anyatovat,* dry eyes.

Medicines required

Medicated oil or *ghrita* as per the requirement.

Materials required

Abhyanga table, *udad* and *yava* flour, cotton, bowls, heater and spoons.

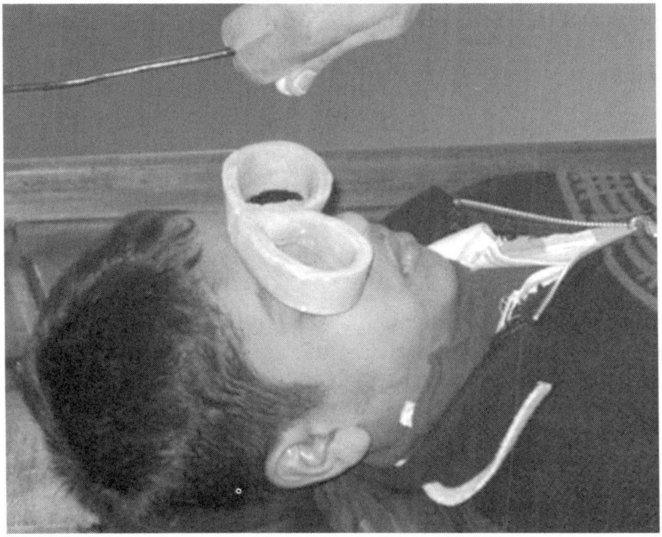

Figure 2.13: *Akshi tarpana*

Preparation

The patient should be purified as per the requirement by *vamana, virechana* or *nasya* or all.

Procedure

After that properly prepared black gram flour shall be applied around eyes so that a pool with a height of about 2 *angula* is created. *Ghrita* or oil shall be heated in hot water bath. This *ghrita* or oil shall be filled when lukewarm into the pool created earlier with eyes closed. The patient should be told to open and close the eyes slowly. This should be repeated till the time of treatment is completed. After this, oil or *ghrita* shall be removed from the lateral corner of the pool or with the help of cotton. After this treatment, the patient should avoid looking directly into the light or towards sky.

Duration of akshi tarpana according to diseases

- In *vartma roga* - 100 *matra*
- In *sandhi roga* - 300 *matra*
- In *sita roga* - 500 *matra*
- In *asita roga* - 700 *matra*
- *Drishti roga* - 800 *matra*
- *Adhimantha* - 1000 *matra*

- *Vataja roga* – 1000 *matra*
- *Pittaja roga* – 600 *matra*
- Healthy people – 600 *matra*

Signs and Symptoms of Samyak Tarpana
Eyes of the patient become light and are able to see in light properly and if it is not done properly, opposite signs will appear like heaviness in eyes, blurred vision, etc.

Karna Purana

It is the method where medicated *sneha* is instilled and filled in the ears. It can be done as a part of daily regimen for prevention of diseases and also as cure for many ailments.

Materials required
Abhyanga table, *gokarna yantra*/dropper, cotton, pillow, towels, spoon, bowl, stove.

Medicines required
Prescribed oil/*ghee*/*swaras,* etc.

Procedure
After proper anointment and sudation done around the ear, the patient is asked to lie in lateral position. The prescribed *sneha* is then filled with the help of *gokarna*/*dropper* and kept filled till 100 *matra* in ear diseases, 500 *matra* in throat-related diseases, and 1000 *matra* in *shiroroga*. Same procedure is followed on the other ear as well. At the end of treatment after cleaning the ears, the patient should rinse the mouth with warm water. It also improves the hearing capacity and prevents any loss of hearing power.

Uses
- It is beneficial in diseases such as *manyastambha, manyagraha, hanugraha, badhirya, karna nada,* etc.
- It prevents vitiation of *vata dosha* in ears.
- Nourishes ear functions and prevents damage to ear.

Mastishkya

Application of *sneha dravya* or pastes mixed with *sneha* over head for nourishment of *mastishka* (brain) is known as *mastishkya*. It is called as *pottichil* in Kerala. In this procedure, it is necessary to shave the head of the patient to gain the maximum effects of this treatment.

Many references of *mastishkya* can be found according to various *shiroroga* in *sushruta samhita*. It is also called as *thalam*. It is an easier means of *shirolepa*. It is also helpful in preventing the harmful effects of *svedana* procedures like *patrapinda sveda* and *shalishashtika pinda sveda*. It serves the purpose of protecting *shiro-marma* when done during other sudation procedures. Its procedure is as under:

Medicines required
Amlaki churna, buttermilk, prescribed oils.

Materials required
Stove, stool, plates, bowls, cotton, gauze, towels

Procedure
The patient is anointed and made to sit comfortably on a stool. The paste of *amlaki churna* and buttermilk is heated till it is lukewarm. The paste is applied properly on the head and a bandage is applied over it and around forehead so that there is no downward leakage of the substance. This paste is removed after the completion of prescribed duration or at the end of other procedure.

Alternative medicines
Eladi churna, rasnadi churna, panchagandha churna, etc. can be used with or instead of *amlaki churna* in preparation of paste.

Uses
- It works as a protective measure for *shiromarma* in many treatments.
- It improves eyesight.
- It is helpful in curing diseases like insomnia, sinusitis and headaches.
- Nourishes hair and prevents hair fall and premature greying.

Taloptichill

It is a special type of thalam procedure which is famous in South India. It is also known as pottichill. It is very effective in various types of psychosomatic disorders. In this treatment, the paste which is applied over the head is covered with leaves, which give the effect of mild form of *svedana*. It is done early in the morning on empty stomach patient.

Medicines required
Amlaki, buttermilk, prescribed oil, water and lotus leaves/leaves of the desired plant.

Materials required
Bowls, heater, spoons, gauze, cotton, etc.

Preparation

Take 16 *tola amlaki* and mix it with 32 *tola* buttermilk prepared from cow's milk and 32 *tola* of water. Heat it till the liquid part of the mixture gets evaporated, after that grind this mixture till it is soft to touch, i.e. in the paste form and care shall be taken to not to add any liquid or water to it.

Procedure

The patient is advised to be empty stomach and clear of the natural urges when this treatment is done. If possible, the head shall be shaved. Light *abhyanga* of head and body is done followed by sudation with warm towels. A bandage is tied around the forehead to prevent any material flowing down to the face or eyes. The prepared mixture is taken when still warm and applied over the shaved head of the patient, making a layer which is about 1/4th to 1/3rd inches thick. The layer is formed carefully applying it to the front sides and back of head leaving a small portion in the *brahma randhra* region open. The prescribed oil is then poured into this central portion. After this, paste is covered with leaf of desired plant/ lotus leaf carefully so that it covers all except the central open portion in which oil is filled. This can be kept for one to one and a half hours. After that the pack is removed and wiped, followed by light *shirobhyanga*. It can be done for 7–14 days. At the end of the treatment, *rasnadi churnam* is applied on the vertex **(Figs 2.14A to C)**.

Uses

- It gives nourishment to the brain and prevents different type of *vataja shiroroga* and enhances memory.
- It is useful in various types of skin diseases.
- It gives strength to eyesight and induces natural sleep.
- Can be used in *sannipatika jvara, nasagata raktasrava.*
- It is also useful in cases of mental retardation.

Gandusha

Gandusha means *mukha purnam,* i.e. filling of the mouth. It is a procedure in which oil/decoctions are held in mouth without making any movements. It is classified into four types according to the therapeutic effects:

Snigdha gandusha

In this, oil treated with *madhura, amla* and *lavana rasa* medicines is used for *gandusha*. It is indicated in *vataja mukharoga.*

Shamana gandusha

Liquid medicines with *sheeta virya* and *pittashamaka rasa* are used for *gandusha*. It is indicated in *pittaja mukharoga.*

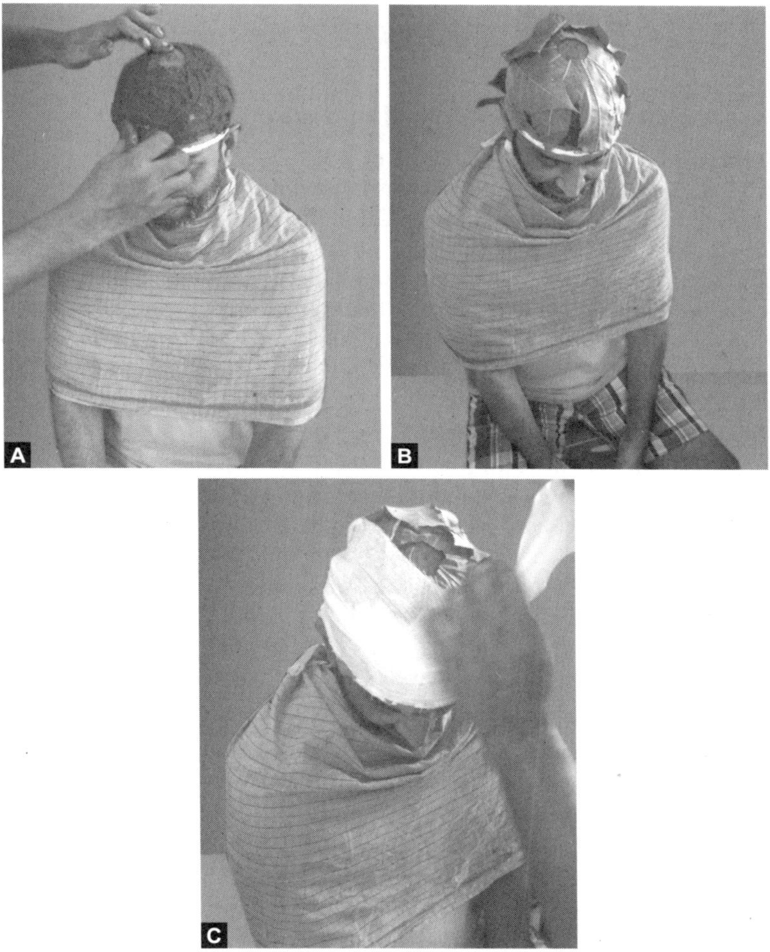

Figures 2.14A to C: Various steps of *Taloptichill*

Shodhana gandusha

In this, warm irritant oil or liquids which are *ushna* in *virya* and have *kaphaghna rasa* are used for *gandusha*. It is indicated in *kaphaja mukharoga*.

Ropana gandusha

In this, oil or liquids prepared from *ushna* medicines are used for *gandusha*. It is indicated in *mukhaja vrana*.

Medicines required
Prescribed oils/decoctions/liquids

Materials required
Abhyanga table, bowls, chair, spoon, towels, stove, spittoon.

Procedure
The patient is given face massage followed by sudation. After this, the patient is allowed to sit on the chair and given the medicine—oil or decoction while lukewarm to hold in mouth without gargling. The medicine shall be filled to the maximum capacity of the patient. After holding the medicine in mouth for the desired period, the patient is allowed to spit out the medicine and then gargle with warm water. The maximum duration is recognized by the symptom, *kaphapurnasyata, nasasrava* and *netrasrava.*

Uses
It gives strength to mandible and improved voice. It prevents dryness of mouth and lips. Increases stability of teeth and gums and prevents caries and toothache. It can be used as part of daily regimen as a preventive measure. But it is contraindicated in persons suffering from *visha, murcha, mada, shosha, raktapitta, kshina rogi* and below the age of 5 years.

Kavala

Kavala is a procedure in which medicated oil is filled into the mouth till half of its capacity and followed by gargles after that. It is having the properties which are similar to *gandusha* in many ways and is of four types:

Snehi kavala
Oil or decoctions which are indicated in *vataroga* are used.

Prasadi kavala
Oil or sweet cool liquids which are indicated in *pittaja roga* are used.

Shodhi kavala
Warm irritant oils or liquids are used. It is indicated in *kaphaja mukharoga.*

Ropana kavala
Oils or liquids prepared from *madhur, katu, tikta* and *kashaya rasa* medicines are used for *kavala*. It is indicated in *mukhaja vrana.*

Medicines required
Prescribed oils/decoctions/liquids

Materials required
Abhyanga table, bowls, chair, spoon, towels, stove, spittoon.

Procedure
The best time for *kavala* is said to be early in the morning. After face massage and light sudation, the patient is made to sit on the chair and liquid medicine given. The warm medicine is filled in the mouth till half capacity and gargles are done for desired time. After gargling, the patient is allowed to spit out the oils and other liquids. Cleanse the mouth by gargling with lukewarm water. The signs and symptoms of completion of *kavala* are similar to *gandusha*.

Uses
It gives strength to mandible and improved voice. It prevents dryness of mouth and lips. Increases stability of teeth and gums and prevents caries and toothache. It can be used as part of daily regimen as a preventive measure. It also helps in curing pains of the sides of neck. It prevents dryness of throat and cracking of lips.

Snehavgahan

It means submerging a part or whole of the body in *sneha dravya*.

Medicines required
Prescribed oil/decoction

Materials required
Bowls, heater, *avgaha yantra*

Preparation
The oil is warmed enough so that it won't be cold but kept cool enough so that the patient will not get burnt.

Procedure
The warmed oil is filled in the tub and the patient is asked to sit inside with body submerged in the *sneha* to the point needed. If it is being done for *sarvanga,* then the patient should be submerged till neck in the *sneha dravya*.

Uses
Snehavgaha gives strength to all the body parts. It is helpful is conditions where medicine is not acting through internal route and is difficult to apply externally. It helps in healing of internal injuries caused by blunt impact.

Sthanik Vasti

It is a special type of local procedure which resembles the process of *shirovasti*. It can be applied on various parts of the body and has many names depending on where it is applied. It directly gives relief in painful conditions and many other diseases. The word *vasti* or *basti* in this procedure means to stay or cover and to dwell. It is achieved with the help of *masha pishti*. It can be perceived as local *snigdha sveda*. Various types of *sthanik vasti* and the site of their application are as follows:

Greeva/manya vasti: Applied on cervical region of spine and helps in curing cervical ailments **(Fig. 2.15)**.

Prishtha vasti: Applied on dorsal region of spine and helps in curing various diseases of this part.

Kati vasti: Applied on lumbosacral region and helps in curing diseases like sciatica, lumbar spondylitis, etc. **(Fig. 2.16)**.

Janu vasti: Applied on knee joints and nourishes them. Also cures arthritis, osteophytes and loose calcified bodies **(Fig. 2.17)**.

Uro/hridaya vasti: Applied on cardiac region of thorax and helps in curing diseases of this part.

Medicines required
Prescribed oils/*kuzambu*

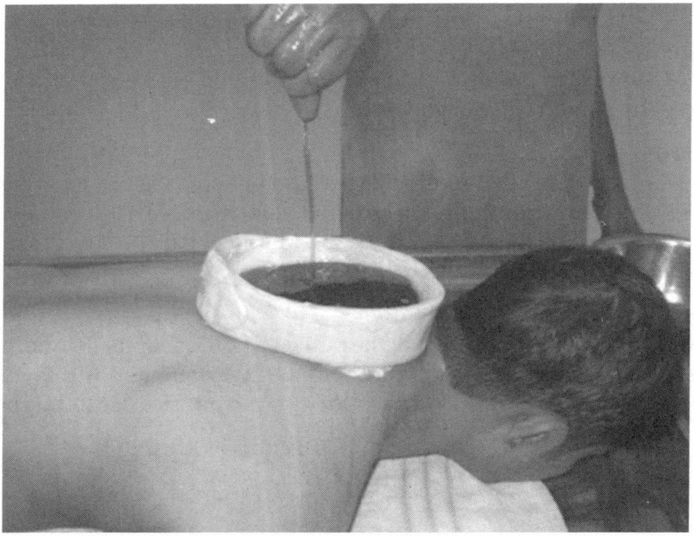

Figure 2.15: *Greeva vasti*

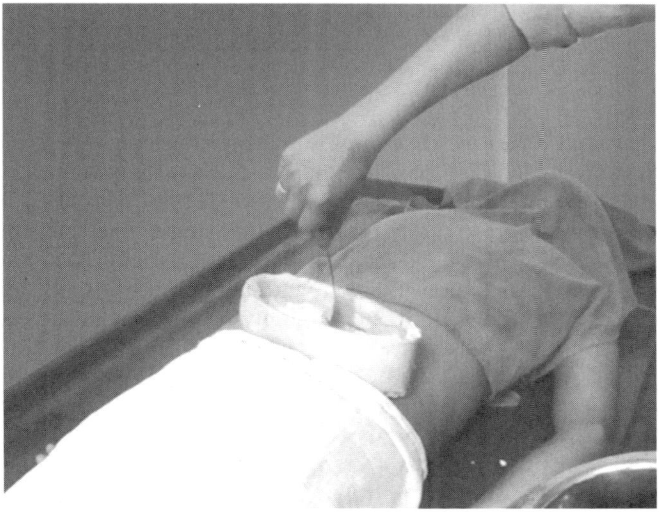

Figure 2.16: *Kati vasti*

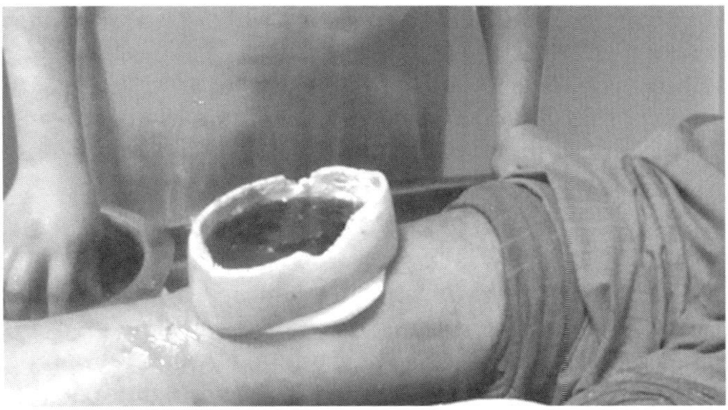

Figure 2.17: *Janu vasti*

Materials required

Bowls, heater, sponge pieces, cotton, *udada* (black gram) and *godhuma* (wheat) flour, steel or plastic rings, if available, water.

Preparation

The oil is warmed enough so that it won't be cold but not so hot, that the patient gets burnt. The part where *vasti* needs to be applied is properly anointed and sedated with *nadi sveda*/hot towels. The water bath is required to be kept heated so that the oils can be heated repeatedly during the procedure.

Procedure

Patient is made to lie down in a comfortable position and draped properly so that only the affected part is exposed. Previously prepared ring of the *udada* (black gram) and *godhuma* (wheat) flour is applied on the part where we need to apply the *vasti*. This ring is fixed properly so that the oils/medicines filled inside will not leak or spill out of it easily. The oil is first filled by pouring it along the boundaries of the ring and when the skin of the patient is completely submerged in the oil, and then we can pour it directly inside. The temperature of oil is continuously maintained at the same level by taking out little amount of oil with the help of a spoon/sponge/cotton and refilling it with warm oil repeatedly. It is important to not to let the skin of the patient come in direct contact of the air till this procedure is complete. This procedure is done for 30–45 minutes depending upon the severity of the disease and can be done for 7/14/21/28 days.

After the treatment is complete and oil is removed and dough too is taken out, the affected part is gently massaged again. Clean the area with hot water and let the patient rest for a while. Precaution should be taken to not to overheat the oil.

Various types of oils which can be used in these treatments are—*Sahacharadi taila, sahacharadi kuzambu, dhavantaram taila, dhanvantaram kuzambu, mahanarayana taila* and *murivenna taila,* etc.

Uses

It is useful in various types of *vatavyadhis* like *greevagata vata, katigata vata, sandhi gata vata, gridhrasi,* blunt injuries, arthritis, spondylitis, disc prolapsed, muscular spasms, osteophytes, calcified loose bodies and some cardiac diseases. It is *balya* and *vataghna* in properties and various types of oils can be used to achieve the desired results.

These therapies work by improving the blood circulation of the affected part. The medicines along with the oil are absorbed and digested with the help of *bhrajaka pitta* and act directly on the affected part. It also soothes the muscular tissue by the heat present in oils.

Sneha Karmukatva

Mode of action of snehana can be studied in two ways—one is its action as *poorvakarma* to *shodhana* and the second is the mode of action as *pradhana karma* in itself.

Mode of action of *snehana as pradhana karma* is as under:

- Pacifying the vitiated *vata dosha*.
- Melting the excessive *dosha* lodged in the parts of the body which are having *kha vaigunya*.
- Increasing the digestive power of not only *jathragni* but all the *dhatvagnis* too.
- Cleanses the *koshtha* and expels all the toxins (*mala*) from body.
- Initiates the development of new *dhatus* thus increasing the strength of the body.
- Improves *varna*
- Delays the aging process which provides longevity

Sneha karmukta as a *poorvakarma* has been described by the classics by citing a few examples which are as under:

- If the walls of an utensil are properly anointed and are filled with water and turned over, not a single drop of water will be left sticking to inside. Similarly, after proper *snehana*, all the *doshas* start moving from the extremities and are collected in *koshtha* and thus can be expelled by *shodhana*.
- The way a cloth when merged in water absorbs some and, on being squeezed, retains just a bit but expels out most part. Similarly, the body absorbs some part of the *sneha* according to the digestive power and expels out the rest.

According to our understanding, the mode of action of *sneha* in *poorvakarma* involves all the processes which classics try to cite by different examples. The *sneha* when given in steady quantities over days gradually goes to all the *dhatus* and breaks the *dosha dushya sammurchana*, and as the center of gravity of the body is *koshtha* (also referred to as *mahanimna* in some texts) all the *dosha*, thus released, start travelling towards the *koshtha* and as all the vessels are properly anointed like the example of the utensil, no part of these *doshas* stays inside them and all the vitiated material is collected in the *koshtha*, which can be expelled through the nearest route which is the main motto of *shodhana chikitsa*.

But it is also important to remember that *svedana* also plays a crucial role in increasing the efficacy of *snehana*.

CHAPTER 3 Svedana

The procedure by which sweating is induced in the body is called as *svedana*. It is also termed as sudation therapy or fomentation therapy.

DEFINITION

It is defined as a procedure which reduces the stiffness of the body, reduces heaviness and cold, and brings out sweat, is called *svedana*. Another definition puts it as the *sagni* or *niragni* procedure; in which heat is given to the *snigdha* patient is *svedana*. *Svedana* is especially useful in diseases caused by vitiated *vata* and *kapha dosha*. It is used as *poorvakarma* as well as *pradhana karma,* especially in *vata* dominant diseases.

The reason behind doing *svedana* after *snehana* is that the *doshas* which have previously been loosened from the *srotosanga* by *snehana,* can be directed by *srotovilayana* to the *koshtha* so that when the time for purification comes, they can be easily expelled through the nearest route.

PROPERTIES OF SVEDANA DRAVYA

Properties of *svedana dravya* are *ushna, tikshna, sara, snigdha, ruksha, sukshma, drava* and *sthira*.

CLASSIFICATION OF SVEDANA

Although there are many ways in which *svedana* is classified but it is essentially of two types as already discussed—*Sagni sveda* and *Niragni sveda* depending upon the fact whether *agni* is to be used or not for the induction of sveda in the body.

- *Niragni sveda:* No direct heat or *agni* is required to induce *sveda*. It is produced indirectly. It is of following ten types:

1. *Vayayama*: Exercising, it is one of the easiest ways of sudation and also nourishes body and improves strength.
2. *Ushna sadana*: Sitting in warm room with thick walls, this warmth is achieved by preventing ventilation and not with the help of any form of heat.
3. *Guru pravarana*: Covering one with heavy woollen clothes.
4. *Kshudha*: Not eating food when feeling hungry also induces *svedana*.
5. *Bahupana*: Drinking liquids especially alcohol in excess quantity.
6. *Bhaya*: Fear, inducing fears leads to sweating. *Bhaya* and *krodha* directly stimulate sympathetic nervous system and induce sweating.
7. *Krodha*: Anger, inducing anger vitiates *pitta* and helps in sweating.
8. *Upnaha*: Poultice, it is included here as there is no direct contact of heat producing substances. It is a kind of localized sweating.
9. *Aahata*: Wrestling with hands, it is also called as *niyuddha*. It induces exertion and thus leads to sweating.
10. *Aatapa*: Sunbath, it is very beneficial in many skin and *vata* disorders.

- *Sagni sveda* is of four major types:
  1. *Tapa sveda*
  2. *Upnaha sveda*
  3. *Ushma sveda*
  4. *Drava sveda*
- *Charakokta* 13 *sveda*: Acharya Charak has described following 13 types of *svedana* procedures, which get included in the above mentioned four types.
  1. *Sankara*
  2. *Prastara*
  3. *Nadi*
  4. *Parisheka*
  5. *Avagaha*
  6. *Jentaka*
  7. *Ashmaghna*
  8. *Karshu*
  9. *Kuti*
  10. *Bhu*
  11. *Kumbhi*
  12. *Koopa*
  13. *Holaka*

SVEDANA YOGYA–AYOGYA

People Who are *Svedana Yogya*

Those suffering from *pratishyaya, kasa, hikka, shvasa, angagaurav, karnashula, manya shula, shirah shula, svarabheda, galagraha, ardita, ekangavata, sarvangavata, pakshaghata, vinamaka, aanaha, vibandha, shukraghata, jrumbha, parshvagraha, prushthagraha, katigraha, kukshigraha, hanugraha, gridhrasi, mutrakrichra, mushkavriddhi, angamarda, padarati, jangharati, janvarati, uru arati, pada janu jangha uru graha, shotha, raballi, aamdosha, shaitya, vepathu, vatakantaka, sankocha, aayasa, stambha, supti*, the one who is to be given *nasya*, those who are eligible for *vasti, vamana* and *virechana*, those whose *shalya* has been removed, ladies after normal delivery, *bhagandar, arsha, ashmari, arbuda, granthi* and *adhyavat.*

When studying the above list, we can classify it into three heads: *vatavyadhi, kaphaja vyadhi* and those who are posted for *shodhana* or *shalya karma.*

People Who are *Svedana Ayogya*

Alcoholic, pregnant ladies, those suffering from *raktapitta, atisar, madhumeha, bhrishta, braghna, sthula, pittaja prameha, trishna, kshudha*, anger, *kamla, udara, urahkshata, urustambha, timira, panduroga, ajirna*, diseases which require *stambhana, gudabhransh* and similar diseases, those who have taken poison, those with alcohol-related diseases, *vidagdha, pittaja prakriti* people, those who have taken milk, alcohol, curd and ladies with active menstruation.

Studying the above list reveals there are three types of people in this, one who are suffering from *pittaja* ailments, secondly those who have a disease in the extreme levels, and third are those who cannot bear the *svedana* procedure as they are too weak.

Here onwards, we will discuss the details of individual *svedana* procedures.

SANKARA SVEDA

It is a procedure in which sudation is given by the required medicines while having them tied in a cloth in the form of *pottali.* Sometimes, it can also be done without having them in a *pottali* form. It is also called as *pinda sveda.* It is of two types, *Snigdha sankara sveda* and *ruksha sankara sveda.*

Snigdha Sankara Sveda

It is done with medicines such as *tila, masha,* rice, etc. and done with the help of *amla drava,* milk, etc. It is beneficial in *vatavyadhis.* Following are a few types of *snigdha sankara sveda* which are in practice:

Shashtika Shali/Shali Shashtika Pinda Sveda

It is famous in South India by the name *navarakizhi.* It is done with the boluses prepared of *navara,* rice, i.e. shali rice. It is very beneficial in various types of *vatavyadhi.* Its procedure is as follows **(Fig. 3.1)**:

Medicines required
Navara rice 400 g, *bala mula kvatha*—2 liters, Cow's milk—2 liters, Prescribed oil/*kuzambu, amlaki* paste.

Materials required
Droni/Abhyanga table, bowls, heater, square cloth pieces 20 × 20 - 8, threads, spatula, steel vessels, plastic apron, and flexible thin plastic scrapper.

Preparation
At firs,t we prepare *balamula kwatha* approx 192 tola. Out of this, half of the *kwatha* is taken out and mixed with equal amount of milk. *Navara* rice is the cleaned and cooked in this mixture of *balamula kawatha*

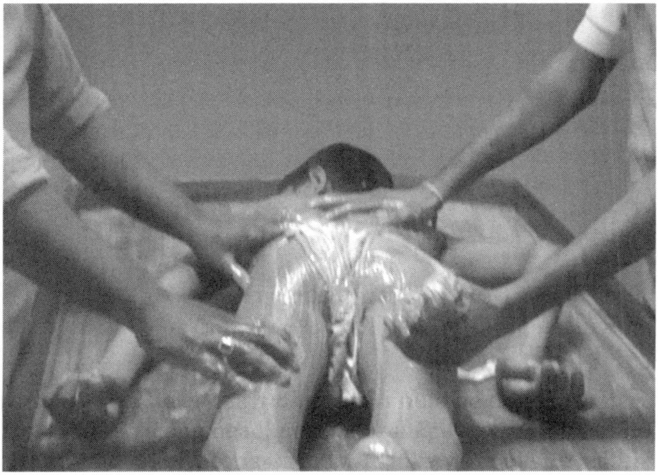

Figure 3.1: *Shashtika shali pinda sveda*

and milk, till the liquid part gets completely evaporated. The prepared mixture is then taken into the eight cloth pieces and pottalis/bolus bundles are prepared out of it in a way that there is enough cloth extending out to hold in the grip. Rest of the *kwatha* and milk is mixed and is heated on low flame to begin the treatment.

After this *amlaki kalka* is prepared to do *taladharana* before this procedure is started. It saves the *shiro-marma* from any damage while this very hot procedure is performed. For this 100 g of *amlaki churna* is mixed with 200 mL takra and heated till liquid part is completely evaporated. After that, it is applied over the head when still lukewarm.

Procedure

At first, whole body of the patient is properly anointed by doing light *abhyanga*. The bolus bundles prepared are kept in the mixture of *balamula kvatha* and milk which is being heated on low flame. They are taken out when warm and slowly applied over the body of the patient. The bundles are used alternately so that there is no chance to let the body cool down while the treatment is being done. It is done continuously for 40–60 minutes for whole body and 15–20 minutes for a part of body. The strokes of the bundles should be circular or oval all over the body. All the seven postures of *abhyanga* can be followed here too. At the end of treatment the paste which is all over the body is gently scraped off and cleansed with hot towel. At the end, remove the *kalka* from the head and clean the scalp too. This procedure can be done for 7, 14, 21 or 28 days according to the requirement.

Uses

- It is useful in various types of *vatavyadhi* especially conditions such as, *shosha, pakshaghata, khanja, pangu, avabahuka,* etc.
- It is also very beneficial in muscular dystrophy and asthma.
- It is also curative in certain types of *raktaja* disorders.

Annalepana

It is a procedure in which the rice prepared such as *shalishashtika pinda sveda* is applied over the body directly similar to the procedure of *upnaha* or *pradeha*. The only difference between *shalishashtika pinda sveda* and *annalepana* is that instead of preparing *pottali*/bundles of rice in cloth pieces, we directly apply the cooked *payasa* over the body. Although similar, *annalepana* is a far more effective treatment when compared to *shalishashtika pinda sveda*. It is famous in Kerala as *navara techirippu*.

Important thing to be kept in mind during the procedure of *pinda sveda* or *annalepana* is to keep a watch on bowel movement. They shall be regular and if there is constipation, it shall be managed accordingly.

Medicines required

Navara rice 400 gms, *bala mula kvatha* - 192 tola, Cow's milk - 2 liters, Prescribed oil/*kuzambu, amlaki* paste.

Materials required

Droni/Abhyanga table, bowls, heater, square cloth pieces 20 × 20 - 8, threads, spatula, steel vessels, plastic apron, and flexible thin plastic scrapper.

Preparation

It is similar to that in *shalishashtika pinda sveda*. After the material is prepared, patient is taken in *droni* and made to lie down properly. Light *abhyanga* is done over the body and then the procedure is started.

Procedure

Lukewarm paste is taken to start the main procedure. The masseurs shall be trained in holding the hot paste in the hands or the treatment will not be done properly. This warm paste is gently applied all over the body and kept in place for a while. This paste is kept till it gets cold, and then it is removed. This can be applied to one part of the body in localized diseases or all over the body below neck in conditions pertaining to whole body. As the contact is more, the resulting *brihana karma* is also more.

The paste is removed by scraping with coconut leaves or with towels soaked in hot water. At the end of treatment, *samvhana* with oil is done. After this treatment, patient should take rest for some time.

Uses

It is beneficial in *vataja* diseases such as spasms, stiffness, weakness, debility, muscular dystrophy. It is also beneficial in hypertension and certain skin diseases.

Patra Pottali/Patrapinda Sveda

It is a variety of *pinda sveda* in which different types of leaves are fried with specific oils and material and bolus bundles are prepared and *pinda sveda* given. It is useful in various types of *vatavyadhi*.

Medicines required

Grated leaves of *Eranda* (Ricinus Communis), *Arka* (Calotropis Gigantiea), *Amlika* (Tamarindus Indica), *Nirgundi* (Vitex Negundo),

Dhattura (Datura Metal), Fried powder of *Shatava* (Peucedanum Graveolens) and *Methika* (Trigonella Foenumgraecum), Scrapings of *Coconut* (Coconut Nucifera), *Nimba* (Azadirachta Indica), *Taila* and *Lemon*.

Materials required

- Two pieces of clean cloth - 45 × 45 cm
- Thread
- Earthen pan
- Stove
- Prescribed oil
- Towel/napkins

Preparation

All the medicines are taken together in a pan and mixed with *nimba taila* and heated mildly. The fried mixture is divided into two equal parts and transferred into the cloth pieces, and fasten with threads to form two balls **(Figs 3.2A to I)**.

Out of the two balls thus prepared **(Fig. 3.3)**, keep the one ball in vessel over low heat for a few minutes. In order to avoid charring of the balls, the vessel is applied with castor/*nimba*/prescribed oil.

Procedure

Warm oil/*Kuzhambu* is applied over the affected part of the patient's body. The warm ball is taken and massaged on affected part with gentle force. As soon as the ball that is on the body starts getting cold it is replaced with the warm one from the vessel. Care shall be taken to not to overheat these *pottali*.

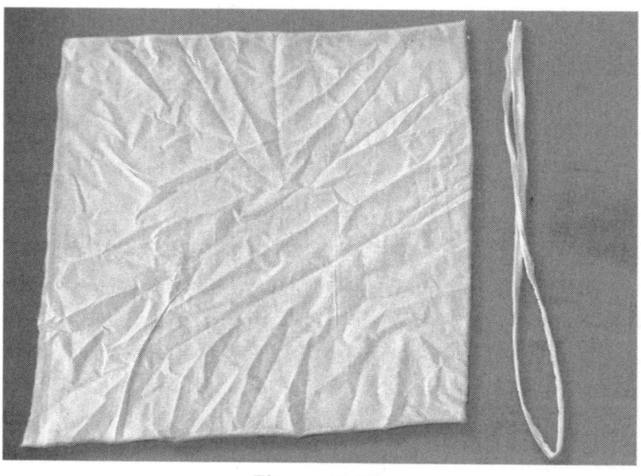

Figure 3.2A

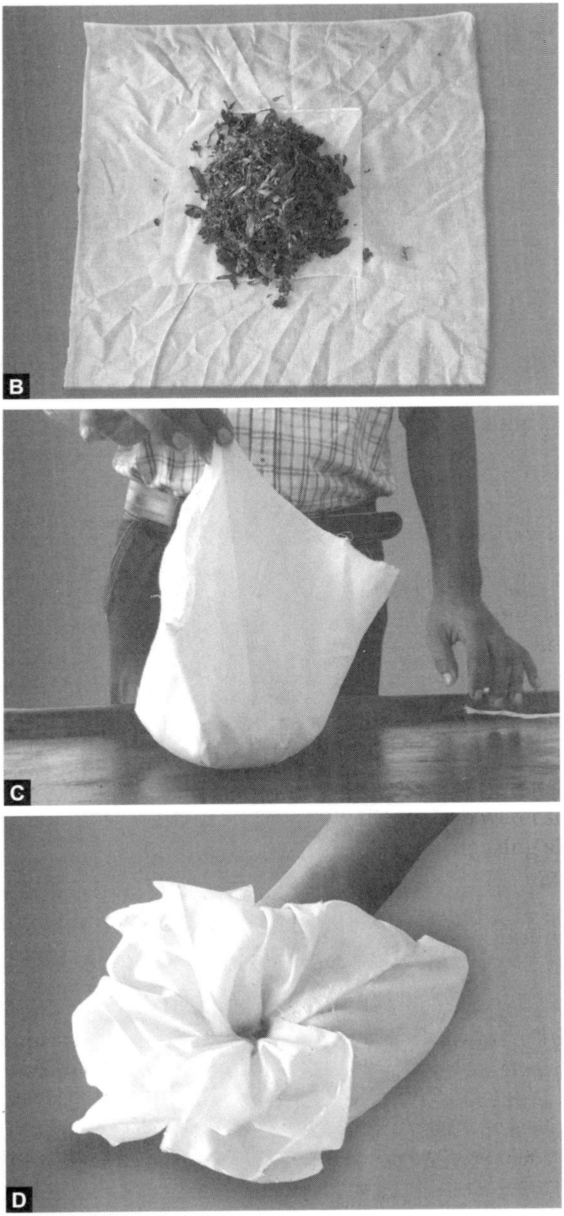

Figures 3.2B to D

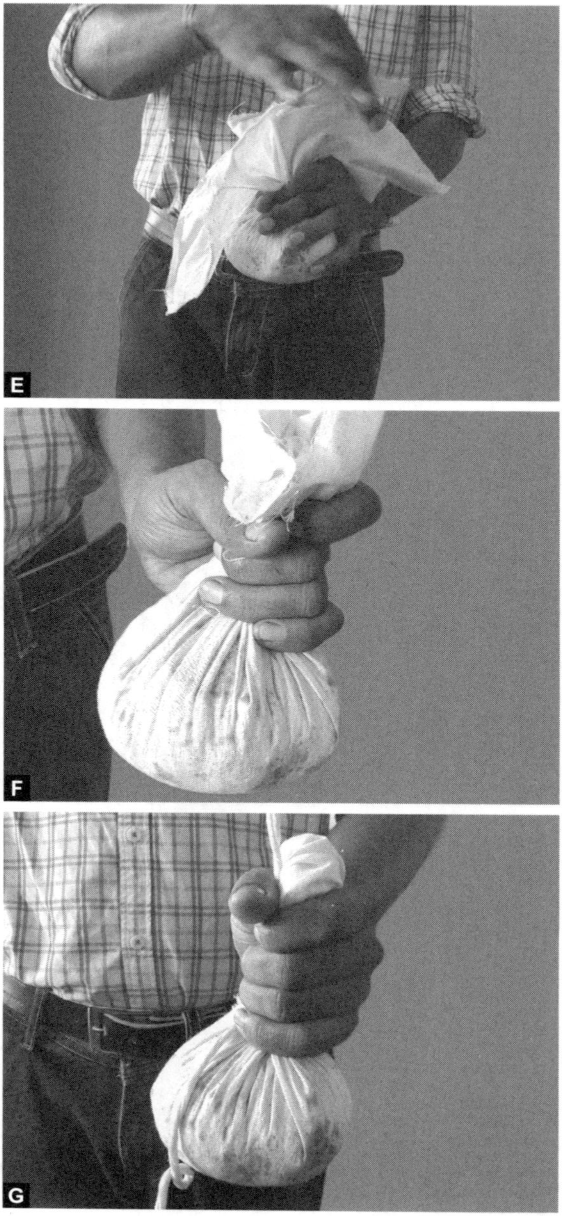

Figures 3.2E to G

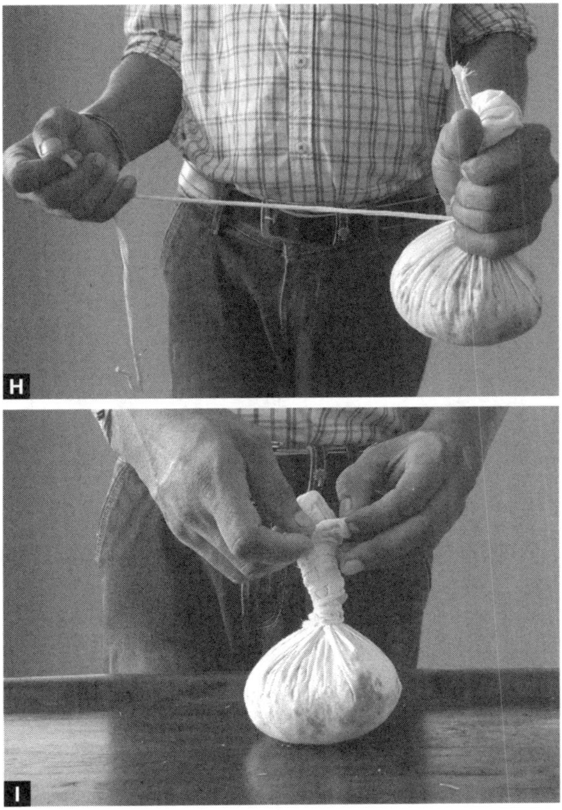

Figures 3.2H and I

Figures 3.2A to I: Prepration of *Patra Pottali/Patrapinda*

This process should be repeated without interruptions for 45–60 minutes time. After the massage is complete, clean the body parts by wiping off the extra oil by a napkin/clean towel. Immediate bathing is not advisable **(Fig. 3.4)**.

Uses

- It is a light variety of *pinda sveda.*
- It is very effective in *kaphaja* diseases.
- It is used with success in bronchitis and asthma.
- It is useful in joint pain, spondylosis, neuromuscular disorders and skin problems, etc.

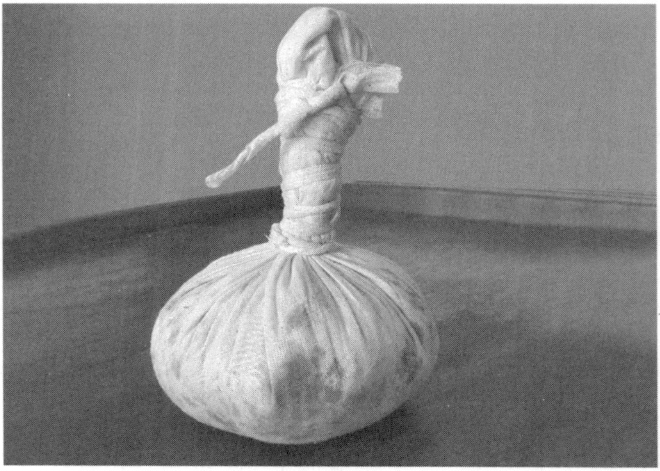

Figure 3.3: Prepared *Pottali*

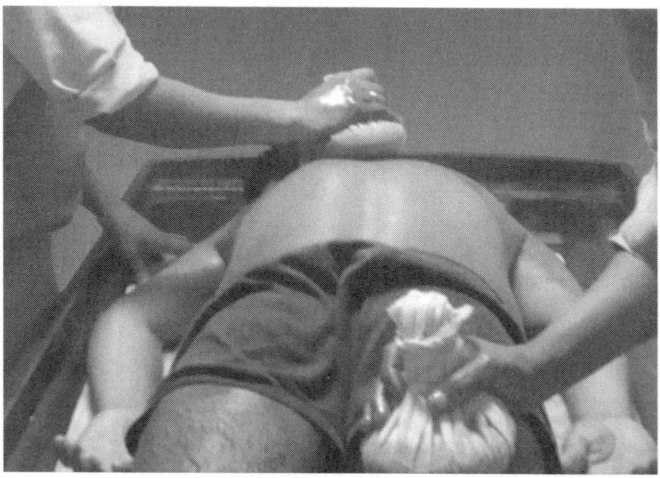

Figure 3.4: *Patrapinda sveda*

Ruksha Sankara Sveda

It is done with dry feces of cow, camel, horse, etc., *valuka*, iron ball, etc. It is beneficial in *kaphaja* and *amavata* like diseases. Its main purpose is to induce *rukshana karma*, which is essential in treatments of *amanjaya* and *kaphaja* disorders **(Fig. 3.5)**.

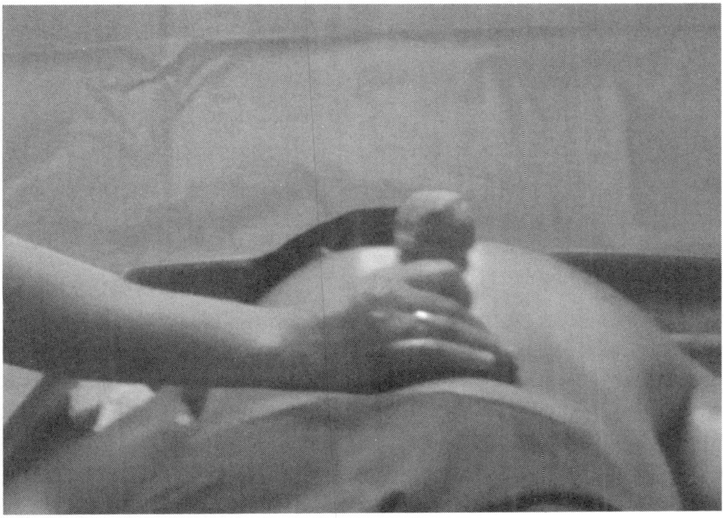

Figure 3.5: *Ruksha sankara sveda*

Valuka Sveda

It is a variety of *ruksha sankara sveda* and is done with the help of bundles prepared of sand. It is very easy to be done and can be performed anywhere and at any given point of time. It is especially useful in *kaphaja* diseases and various *ama dosha* conditions.

Medicines required
Medicated oil, if required

Materials required
Sand, cloth pieces 18 × 18 – 2, stove, earthen pan

Preparation
At first the required quantity of sand is taken and any stones and other materials not required, removed from it. The sand is heated in the pan till it is warm enough, care shall be taken to not to overheat the sand. It is then taken in the cloth pieces and proper bundles prepared so that the sand does not leak out.

Procedure
If the patient is advised then light application of oil on the affected part shall be done. After that this heated bundles of sand are slowly pressed on the affected part, and if it is being done on the whole body,

then slowly the process is repeated all over. This procedure can be done for 30 to 60 minutes and can be repeated more than once a day, if required.

Uses
It is beneficial in curing *amavata* and other similar *vatavyadhi* which have *samavastha* or have *kapha dosha* in addition to *vata*. It is also useful in painful and edematous conditions.

Churna Pinda Sveda

It is similar *valuka pinda sveda* in the meaning that is applied dry over the body. The bundles or *pottali* are prepared from various herbal powders and its benefits are similar to *valuka pinda sveda*. It is also a *rukshana* procedure. The only difference between the two is that it imparts effects of the medicines along with dry heat as given in *valuka pinda sveda*. It is famous in South India by the name *Podikizhi*.

Medicines required
Fine powders of *methika, shatapushpa, kulattha, devadaru, shweta eranda, kola, haridra, rasna, tila, jatamansi. Saindhava lavana* and *nimba* taila are also required.

Materials required
Abhyanga table, cloth pieces, thread, frying pan, towels and stove.

Preparation and procedure
It is similar to the other *pinda sveda* procedures in which a *pottali* is prepared from the medicines and sudation is done by heating the *pottali* repeatedly. This can be done for 45 minutes a day and can be done for 7 to 21 days.

Uses
It is useful in *sama* and *kaphanubandhi vatavyadhi* like *amavata*. It can also be used in spondylitis, obesity, *gridhrasi* and other neurological disorders.

Another variety of churna pinda sveda famous in Northern India
There is a variety of *churna pinda sveda* which is performed similarly but with a different combination of medicines which is famous in North India. The medicines required for this treatment are *katphala, ajwain, masha, erandabija, saindhava lavana, alasi, binola, rasona, black tila*. It is very beneficial in all types of *vatavyadhi* and gives good result in painful and edematous conditions with immediate effect.

PRASTARA SVEDA

It is a type of *svedana* where a person is laid on a bed of stone which is covered with dry rice/wheat/pulses, etc. It is also known as *sanstara sveda*.

Medicines Required

Medicated oil, if required.

Materials Required

A stone of size 6' × 2'6" and two feet high which can be used as a bed, silk cloths, 7' × 3' – 2 pcs, wheat/rice/*krushra*/*payasa*, etc. as indicated for giving sudation, blanket.

Preparation

Patient is well-anointed before the procedure.

Procedure

The stone is first covered with one silk cloth and after that the sudation material is spread over it when still hot; it is then again covered with the second silk cloth piece. The patient is then made to lie on this and covered from top also with the help of a blanket. It is important to take care that the patient does not get burnt during this procedure. It is even better if this procedure can be done in a *nivata sadan*, i.e. a room which is devoid of ventilation.

Uses

It is useful mainly in *vatavyadhi* like *katishula, prishthashula, parshvashula, shronishula, gridhrasi, prishtha-kati sankocha, khalli,* etc.

NADI SVEDA

It is a type of *vashpa sveda* (steam) which is given with the help of a special *yantra* called as *nadi sveda yantra*. *Nadi* means tube-like structure. It is especially useful when we need to give steam to a particular part of body, i.e. *ekanga svedana* can be performed by this procedure easily. It can be performed by decoctions of medicines, *mansarasa* of various animals or especially prepared milk which is also called as *ksheerabala* **(Fig. 3.6)**.

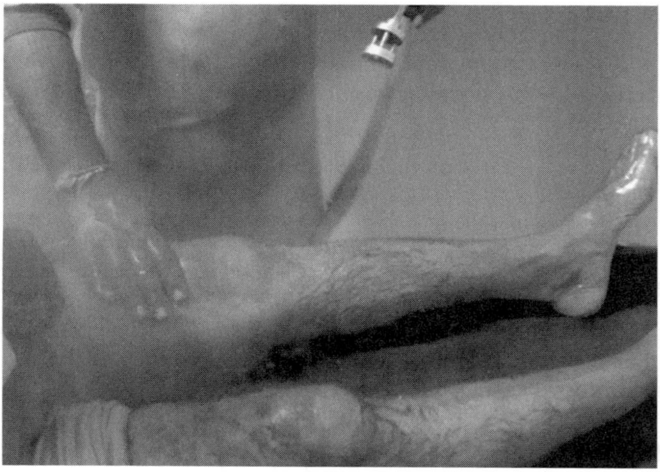

Figure 3.6: *Nadi sveda*

It is important to take adequate length of the tube or pipe to avoid any burns over skin of the patient.

Medicines Required

Decoction of the prescribed medicine and prescribed oil.

Materials Required

Heater, bowls, pan, cooker or steam generator, 6' long rubber pipe which can tolerate high temperatures.

Preparation

At first the decoction of the prescribed medicine is prepared.

Procedure

The decoction is filled in the cooker (this is how the *nadi sveda* is given in the present era, texts give a different detail according to the material and technology present at that time) and kept on stove or heater. The pipe is then attached to the place where whistle is normally attached; the pipe shall be bent or be circulated and not kept straight so that the steam will not come out with the pressure. It is advisable to hold the pipe a bit behind the opening with the help of a cloth. The steam is then given carefully and care is taken that the water drops coming out with the steam will not fall on the patient and burn his skin.

Uses

It is useful in localised stiffness and pains. Especially in conditions such as *kati gata vata, kati shula, janu shula, prishtha shula, manya shula, manya stambha,* etc.

SARVANGA VASHPA SVEDA

It is the second variety of *vashpa sveda,* in which the steam is given to whole body, whereas in *nadi sveda,* it is given to a particular part only. It can be given in a box and be arranged in two postures sitting or laying down **(Fig. 3.7)**.

Medicines Required

Decoction of the prescribed medicine or hot water.

Materials Required

Sarvanga vashpa svedana yantra either sitting or laying down type, towels, cooker or steam generator, wet towels.

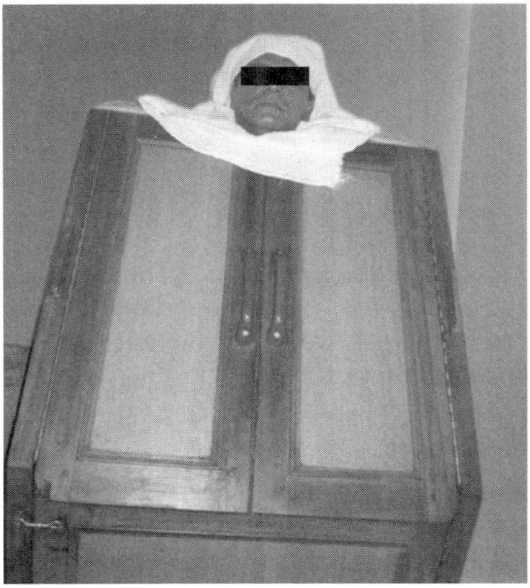

Figure 3.7: *Sarvanga vashpa sveda*

Preparation

At first the patient is given *abhyanga* or any other procedure which is required to be done before *vashpa svedana*. The head of the patient shall be kept out of the table and covered with a wet towel; also he should be given a small amount of water before setting him inside the table.

Procedure

After the necessary preparation, when steam is filled in the box of *svedana yantra*, patient is allowed to move in either sitting or laying down position. The gap under the face is properly covered with towels so that steam will not escape out and head of the patient is covered with a wet towel. The steam can be given till the proper signs of *svedana* are achieved. After this treatment patient shall be rested for about half an hour and allowed bath only after one hour has passed.

Uses

It is beneficial in all types of *vatavyadhis* especially in *gridhrasi, prishthakatigata vata, pakshaghata, mansagata vata.*

DHARA/PARISHEKA SVEDA

Pouring of hot decoctions made up of *vataghna* and *kaphaghna* medicines is called as *dhara sveda*. It is done with the help of a *kumbhi,* which is having a hole in the bottom and the liquid is poured in a continuous stream over the body. In this way, we can give *sarvanga dhara* with the help of decoctions, oils, ghee, milk, etc. **(Fig. 3.8)**.

Pizhichil

It is a very famous type of *sarvanga dhara* in South India. It is done with the help of *vataghna* oils over the body and *droni* is required to get this treatment done properly. Also we need 4 therapists and 2 attendants to perform *pizhichil* on whole body.

Medicines Required

Prescribed medicated oils/*kwatha.*

Materials Required

Droni, dharapatra, sponges, bowl, stove, towels, cotton.

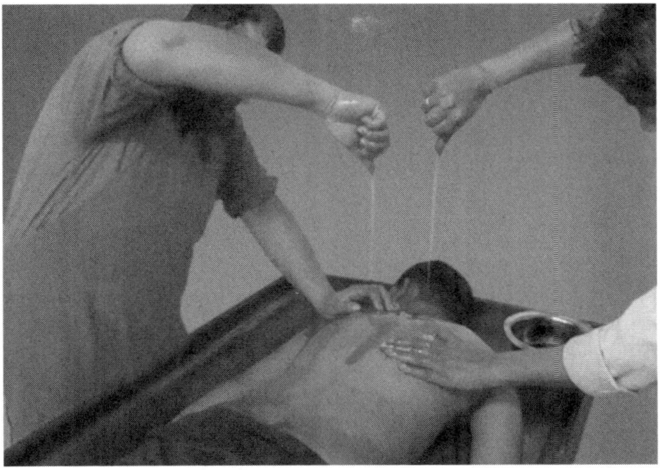

Figure 3.8: *Dhara sveda*

Preparation

The oil is required in a higher quantity in this treatment. The patient is described the procedure in details and then made to lie down on the *droni*.

Procedure

The oil/decoction can be poured over the patient by two methods, one is by using *dharapatra* and other is by using cloth/sponge pieces. The height from which the warm liquids are poured should be around 12 *angula*. From one hand, the *dhara* is poured continuously; while from the other hand, the oil is continuously wiped off the body. While doing *dhara* with the help of a cloth or sponge piece the oil shall be poured with thumbs down posture so that a continuous stream falls over the body through the thumb of therapist. The important thing is to have the therapists trained in holding the cloth pieces which are submerged in hot oil or it will be difficult to complete the procedure. Also one shall be confirming repeatedly, if the oil is not too hot or else the patient can have burn marks. The oil which gets collected at the base of *droni* is recollected and used again after being warmed. This procedure can be done for 30 to 45 minutes for 7, 14, 21 or 28 days.

In this procedure, the milk is changed every day, oil is changed on every third day and so in *dhanyamla*. Oil is kept safe after being used for 1–3 days and then changed and the oil used from 4–6 days is mixed with the previously kept oil and *dhara* is done on the seventh day with this mixture, so on and so forth.

It is important to follow the *parihara kala* for the similar number of days for which *pizichil* is done. Care shall be taken to avoid cold and old food and atmosphere. It is important to follow brahmacharya during this procedure's duration and *parihara kala*.

Uses

- It is helpful in curing diseases such as *gulma, anaha, bhagandara, vrana, tuni, pratituni, shula, abhighata, udavarta, pakshaghata, mudhavata, vidhradhi*, etc.
- It imparts strength to all body organs and improves *oja* and *varna*.
- It is *vrishya*.
- Improves the capacity of all *indriya* and also slows downaging.
- It is also useful in patients suffering from *apatantraka*.
- It is helpful in various gynecological disorders, especially in ladies who are not able to undergo a normal labor. In these patients pizichil is started when 9th month of pregnancy begins, and shall be done for 2 to 3 weeks or till delivery, whichever is earlier.

Dhanyamladhara

It is a special type of *shirodhara* which is done by *dhanyamla*. In this procedure, *dhara* is performed by using vinegar-like preparation made with cereals (*dhanya*). It is a type of *rukshana karma* and comes under *drava sveda*. *Dhanyamla* is also known as *kanjika*.

Medicines Required

Dhanyamla, Medicated oil, *Rasnadi choornam*

Materials Required

Droni, towels, bowls, gauze, cloth pieces

Preparation

For preparation of *dhanyamla*, we require different cereals as under, raw *navara* rice, *kulattha, tina* rice, *varak* rice, sliced lime, dry ginger powder and *ajwain*. All these items are bundled in separate clothes and kept in a large vessel. Adequate amount of water is filled into this vessel and the mouth of this earthen vessel is closed with a cloth. The vessel is then heated with a constant fire at a steady temperature and from 8th day the *dhanyamla* can be used as required.

Procedure

After doing light *abhyanga*, patient is made to lie in the *droni*. The *dhanyamla* is kept heated at a standard temperature and the procedure is done similar to that in pizhichil, only the pressure shall not be applied over the skin. This procedure can be done in the seven positions of *abhyanga* and is done for 45 minutes in one sitting. It can be continued for seven days. After *dhara*, patient is dried properly and rested. *Rasnadi churnam* is applied on *talam* to protect *shiro-marma*.

Uses and Benefits

It is indicated in *vatarakta, amavata*, obesity, burning sensation all over the body (*daha*), pakshaghata and *vatavyadhi* having *kaphanubandha*.

AVAGAHA SVEDA

Avagaha means submerging the body. It is done with the help of *vatahara* decoctions, oils, ghee, *mansarasa*, hot water, etc. The patient is prepared by *abhyanga*, if required.

Materials Required

Avagaha yantra, heater, steel bowls, towels, cotton sponge pieces, big spoons.

Medicines Required

Vatakaphagna oil or prescribed oil/*kashaya*.

Preparation

The oil is heated till it is lukewarm, and is filled in the *avgaha yantra*. Patient is properly anointed before the treatment is started with the prescribed oil.

Procedure

After the patient is properly anointed, he is asked to sit in the tub filled with the decoction/oil of choice till neck-deep/waist-deep according to the requirement of the treatment. The oil is continuously taken out and refilled in small quantities to maintain the temperature. Some texts advise that the body shall be submerged in the warm liquids to the level 6 *angula* above *nabhi*. It can be done till 1 *muhurta*, 4 *muhurta* or till sweating starts.

Uses

- It helps in treating diseases such as *ashmari, shula, kati shula, kati prishthagata vata, gridhrasi, sandhigata vata, vinam*, etc.
- It is also beneficial in treating *arsha* and *bhagandara* like conditions.
- It imparts strength to spinal cord and lower back.

JENTAKA SVEDA

It is a special type of sudation which is done in a especially prepared room which should be close to a water body. This room is called as *kutagara*. The texts give great details regarding construction of this *kutagara* which will be discussed here **(Fig. 3.9)**.

Construction of *Kutagara*

It is constructed in a round shape and close to a water body, preferably in east or north of the city/town. The gate of this house shall be in the north or east direction. This room shall be 24 feet wide and 16 feet high. There shall be plenty of small windows in the walls of this room and a platform shall be constructed at around the wall from one end of gate to the other. At the center of this room, there shall be a fireplace of size 6 feet by 6 feet (or height of the patient). It shall be filled with the right kind of wood.

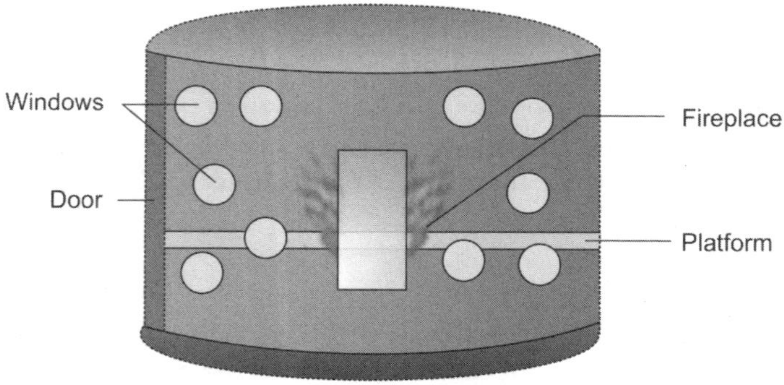

Figure 3.9: *Jentaka sveda kutagara*
(For color version, see Plate 1)

Materials Required

Kutagara as mentioned above, towels.

Medicines Required

Prescribed oil for *abhyanga*, wood of prescribed medicine.

Preparation

The patient shall be anointed properly with the prescribed oil and the fire started in the fireplace which is situated at the centre of the *kutagara*. He shall be educated to lay down on the slab prepared around the room with the wall. He shall change the position when lying down as and when he requires according to his comfort. He shall also be educated to not to leave the support of this slab even, if he is suffocating or facing dehydration and shall come outside with the support of this slab only, or else he may fall unconscious somewhere in the center of the room.

Procedure

After the fire is started and the room is heated enough, the patient who has been anointed already shall be taken inside the room. The patient shall be covered with a cloth when being taken inside and reassured about the treatment. When the patient feels that his body is sweating properly and the stiffness, etc. symptoms have reduced, then he shall come out while taking the support of the slab. This room can be used to give sudation to more than one patient at a time. After the treatment is complete, one shall take rest for about 45 minutes to 60 minutes and then take bath/parisheka with lukewarm water.

Uses

It is useful in all types of *vatavyadhi*, but care shall be taken while selecting the patients that they shall be able to follow the instructions properly and shall not be physically disabled.

It is especially beneficial in diseases which induce stiffness, heaviness and other such symptoms.

ASHMAGHNA SVEDA

It is a type of sudation in which a stone bed is used.

Materials Required

Stone piece 6′ × 2′6″ – 1, water, cloth piece – 6′ × 2′6″ – 2, towels, blankets.

Medicines Required

Wood of prescribed medicine, prescribed oil.

Preparation

The wood of the prescribed plants are burnt on the stone bed and when, they are heated enough, the fire is put out after pouring water and the ashes removed. After that a silk cloth piece is spread over the stone.

Procedure

After the cloth piece is spread over the stone, the patient is made to lie over the stone and is covered with a blanket. Sudation in this process is induced through the steam which evaporates from the heated stone after water is poured over it.

Uses

It is beneficial in various types of *vatavyadhis* specially the ones which include *ama* and *kapha dosha*.

KARSHU SVEDA

It is a type of *sveda* in which sudation is done by fumes of *vata-kaphaghna* medicines which are burnt inside a properly created well. A bed made with the help of ropes which help in the fumes to come through it is kept over a well-prepared ditch which is narrow at mouth and wide at base. The patient is well anointed and made to lie on the bed, and is covered with a woollen blanket. The wood of prescribed medicines is burnt inside and the fumes are given to the patient. It is a type of *ruksha sveda*.

KUTI SVEDA

It is also a type of sudation in which a especially prepared room is required to give sudation. The room prepared for this type of procedure does not have any windows **(Fig. 3.10)**.

Construction of *Kuti*

It is constructed in a round, circular shape. The gate of this house shall be in the north or east direction. This room shall not be too big or too small. The walls of this room should not be having any windows. At the center of this room, a bed is kept which is used to lay down the patient.

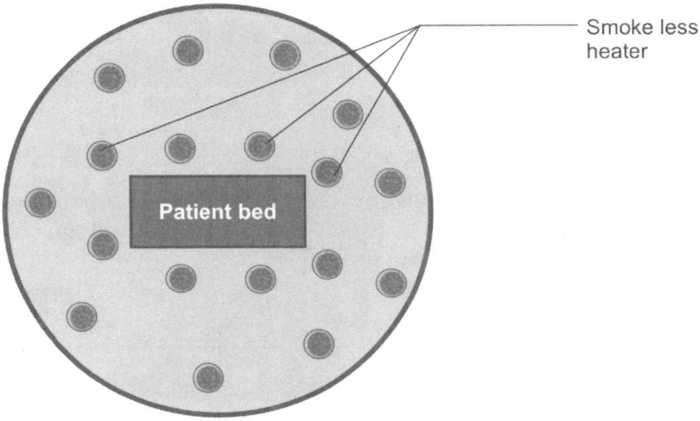

Figure 3.10: *Kuti sveda* (Top view)
(For color version, see Plate 1)

The room is filled with small heaters which use fire to give heat. Care shall be taken that these heaters are not producing any smoke.

Materials Required

Kuti, bed, towels, small heaters for liting up the required wood, and they shall burn smoke free.

Medicines Required

Wood of the required medicine, prescribed oil.

Preparation

The patient is properly anointed before the procedure is started. The wood is burnt inside the small heater/*angithi* while taking care that it is smoke free.

Procedure

The patient who is already anointed properly is taken inside the *kuti* and made to lie down on the bed which is covered with a clean cloth. The small heaters/*angithi*/heaters are already burning while heating the room. Patient is covered with a woollen blanket and is educated about the procedure. When the symptoms of stiffness, etc. are reduced and sweating begins the patient shall come out of the *kuti*.

Uses

It is beneficial in many types of *vatavyadhi*.

Important note: These days this kind of *svedana* can be done in the *sauna* rooms which are easier to construct and install and run on electric heaters and give almost same results

BHU SVEDA

This procedure is similar to the *ashmaghna sveda*, barring the fact that it is done on the floor instead of a stone piece. The wood of the prescribed medicine in burnt in a *nivata sadan*, and then the fire is put off by pouring water and cleaned. A silk cloth is spread on the area and patient is made to lie on it while being covered with the woollen blanket. The uses and properties are similar to *ashmaghna sveda*.

KUMBHI SVEDA

It is a type of *sveda* which is given with the help of a *kumbhi* (pot). This *kumbhi* is buried up to half or one-third part inside the floor. Over this, we keep a bed or rope or a chair which allows the steam to pass through it and is not very high. The *kumbhi* is filled with decoction of the prescribed medicine. After this, we take some iron balls which are heated till red hot and then dipped in the above decoction inside the *kumbhi*. The steam released by this process helps in the sudation.

KUPA SVEDA

'*Kupa*' means a well. It is similar to *karshu sveda*, barring the fact that the depth of the ditch, we dig is twice the height of the bed which is used which comes to about 12 feet deep, 6 feet long and 2 feet 6 inches wide. This ditch is properly cleaned and plastered. After that the ditch is filled with the dry fecal matter of elephant, horse, donkey, cow, etc. This fecal matter is then burnt, and when the fire becomes smoke-free the bed is kept over the ditch and the patient made to lie down after being anointed with the prescribed oil and covered with a blanket. It is a type of *ruksha sveda* and the sudation is also stronger than the *karshu sveda*.

HOLAKA SVEDA

It is a type of sudation in which heat is given by a heater especially prepared. This is of the size which can be adjusted under the bed, and covers the entire base or can be done with the help of small heaters which occupy the underside of the bed and are able to give sudation to whole body of the patient. These heaters are filled with the dry feces of animals like in *kupa sveda* and burnt. The patient is properly anointed and made to lie on the bed of ropes. This procedure is called as *holak sveda*.

Four types of *svedana* procedures described by *Sushruta* and *Vagbhata*.

TAPA SVEDA

It is one of the four types of the *svedana* procedures described by *Sushruta* and *Vagbhata*. *Tapa* means giving heat directly. In this procedure, sudation is done by using the materials such as iron balls, cloth pieces, hands, metals, round-shaped metallic utensils, etc., which are heated directly by fire. It is essentially a *ruksha* kind of *svedana*. Children below 4 months of age shall be given *tapa sveda* by hands, they can also be given *tapa sveda* with the help of cloth piece.

USHMA SVEDA

Ushma means *vashpa* (steam). The procedure in which sudation is given by steam is called as *ushma sveda*. According to descriptions available in *Sushruta Samhita*, the procedures—*jentaka, karshu, kuti, kupa* and *holaka* can be included in this type, along with *nadi* and *sarvanga vashpa svedana*.

UPNAHA SVEDA

The procedure in which sudation is done by tying the *svedana dravya* to the body part is called as *upnaha sveda*. It is an *ekanga sveda*. If *upnaha* is done during daytime, it is removed at night, and if being done at night, it is removed in the next morning. It is indicated in various diseases according to its various types. It is of the following three types as per the descriptions available in Sushruta.

Pradeha

By using the *panchanga* of *vatahara* medicines in the *kalka* form and crushing them with *kanji*, etc *amla dravya* and adding *saindhava lavana* and oil a lepa is prepared which is applied directly over the affected part.

Sankara

Medicines of *kakolyadi gana, eladi gana,* etc., are taken with *tila, alasi, sarshapa,* etc. and crushed in the form of *kalka*. A bolus or *pottali* is then prepared by adding *krushra, payasa, utkarika, veshwara,* etc. to the already prepared *kalka*. Sudation is then done with the help of this bolus.

Bandhana

It is done by using the above-mentioned medicines making them a paste and tying them in a fine cloth, applying it over the affected part and doing a bandage is the third type of *upnaha sveda*.

Salvana Upnaha Sveda

It is a special type of *upnaha sveda* described by *Sushruta* in details under management of *vatavyadhi*. It is done by using medicines described under *kakolyadi gana, eladi gana* or *sursadi gana, vataghna gana,* all the *amla dravyas* (*kanji,* curd, buttermilk, etc.) meat of animals from *anupa desha* and *oudraka* conditions, oil, *ghee, vasa* and *majja* are mixed together and *saindhava lavana* is taken in sufficient quantity. They are heated and applied on the affected part, after which silk/cotton cloth or flesh of cat, rat, mangoose or deer is tied properly. It is done in the diseases such as highly painful conditions, contractures, stiffness, etc.

DRAVA SVEDA

The procedure in which sudation is done with the help of medicated *drava*/liquids is called as *drava sveda*. The medicines which are used in this type of procedure include *vatahara kwatha,* milk, *mansarasa, yusha,* oil, *dhanyamla, ghee, vasa, gomutra,* etc. It is done by two ways—*parisheka* and *avagaha*. The decoctions of *vatahara dravyas* may be sprinkled over the affected part of the body, then the *sveda* is produced, by this method is called as *drava* or *parisheka sveda*. Similarly, the patient can be made to sit in a bathing tub full of warm milk, meat soup or decoction of various drugs to induce fomentation. This is called *avgaha sveda*. This type of sudation is very effective in the management of *arsha, nadi vrana* and *ashmari roga* **(Table 3.1)**.

Table 3.1 Types of *Svedana*

Chaturvdha Sveda According to *Sushruta* and *Vagbhata*	*Sagni Sveda* 13 types According to *Charaka*	*Niragni Sveda*
Tapa ***Ushma/Vashpa*** ***Drava*** ***Upnaha*** Subtypes—*Pradeha, Sankara, Bandhana*	1. *Sankara* 2. *Prastara* 3. *Nadi* 4. *Paisheka* 5. *Avgaha* 6. *Bhu* 7. *Kumbhi* 8. *Kuti* 9. *Jentaka* 10. *Ashmaghna* 11. *Karshu* 12. *Holaka* 13. *Kupa*	1. *Vyayam* 2. *Ushmasadan* 3. *Gurupravarana* 4. *Bahupana* 5. *Ahava* 6. *Atapa* 7. *Kshudha* 8. *Krodha* 9. *Bhaya* 10. *Upnaha*

SIGNS AND SYMPTOMS OF SVEDANA

The signs and symptoms which help us ascertain whether svedana is complete or is done ideally are described in details. It is important to have knowledge of these symptoms to avoid any complications during the treatments.

Samyaka Svinna Lakshana

Shitoparam (cessation of feeling of cold), *shuloparam* (cessation of pain), *stambha nigraha* (reduction of stiffness), *gaurava nigraha* (reduction of heaviness), *mardava* (body becomes soft), sweating is induced, signs and symptoms of disease are pacified, desire of eating or drinking cold products in induced.

Asvinna Lakshana

If sudation is not done properly, then the signs and symptoms which appear are opposite to the symptoms which appear when proper sudation is achieved. They are lack of sweating, feeling cold, heaviness, stiffness, and persistence of painful conditions.

Atisvinna Lakshana

Signs and symptoms of excessive sudation are vitiation of *pitta*, burning sensation in whole body, unconsciousness, tiredness, weak voice, increased pain in joints, appearance of red or black-burning spots, giddiness, *rakta prakopa*, excessive thirst, fever, *klama*, vomiting, etc.

PROCEDURES TO BE GIVEN AFTER SVEDA

After the *svedana* is complete, the most important consideration to be made is purification or *shodhana*. If *svedana* is done for purification, then they shall be performed as per the specified rules. *Vamana* shall be given after one day, *virechana* after 3 days and *vasti, nasya* or *raktamokshana* shall be done immediately, i.e. on the same day.

SVEDANA KARMUKATVA

Svedana acts on the body by performing the following actions:

- It reduces the stiffness (*stambha*) of the body and all the *dhatus*. It induces this by improving the capacity of *dhatvagnis*.
- It reduces the heaviness in body by eliminating and the excessive *kleda* present. It is also induced by stimulation of the muscles and increased circulation inside the vessels.
- It reduces the *shaitya* or feeling of cold.
- It induces sweat, and helps in elimination of toxins with it. It purifies the vessels, muscles and skin. Along with these toxins, *svedana* also expels the *kleda* with sweat. This sweat is induced from the inner *dhatus* as it expels the *kleda* from all of them.
- *Svedana* also imparts liquidity to the *doshas* with the *ushna guna*. These *doshas* which have been softened already by the *snehana* procedure get liquefied and travel easily to the *koshtha*. It is easier for the liquefied *doshas* to travel from the *sukshma srotasas*. It is possible because the *snehana dravya* mixes these *doshas* in it and which melts by the *svedana kriya*.
- *Svedana* along with *snehana* also pacifies the *vata* and channelizes it properly.
- It also induces softness in the organs and muscles, and increases the mobility of all the joints.
- It improves the texture, color, regenerates and beautifies the skin.
- It also improves the *indriyas* and reduces *tandra*.
- *Svedana* also helps in purification of vitiated *doshas* as *poorvakarma*.

CHAPTER

4

Important Medicines for *Snehana* and *Svedana*

In this chapter, a list of important medicines with their indications and modes of use are listed.

TAILA (MEDICATED OILS)

Ayurveda has advised numerous types of oils to be used in various conditions and form a vital part of almost all types of *panchakarma* procedures, more so of *snehana* and *svedana*.

These oils are prepared by using different types of oils as base materials, e.g. *Tila taila* (sesame oil), *kera taila* (coconut oil), *sarshapa taila* (mustard oil), etc. Also, mixture of two bases is used in various formations to give better results, e.g. *Yamaka sneha* which is a mixture of *ghee* and oil, also called as *kuzhambu*.

Some of the important medicated oils and their uses are as below:

Anu Taila

- *Main ingredients: Jivanti, sugandhabala, devadaru, musta, bala*, etc. processed in *shataguna jala* and oil.
- *Indications:* All *vataja, vata-kaphaja* disorders and *shiroroga*.
- *Route of administration*: Through *nasya*
- *Advantage*: It can also be used for promotion of good health as a part of *dinacharya* (healthy regimen).

Asana Bilwadi Taila

- *Main ingredients: Asana, bilva, bala, guduchi*, etc.
- *Indications:* All *netra, karna* and *shiroroga*.
- *Route of administration*: External application or through *nasya/ karnapoorana*
- *Advantage*: Best used for *shalakya tantra*.

Bala Taila

- *Main ingredients: Bala, yashtimadhu, ela, chandana*, etc.
- *Indications:* All *vataja* disorders.
- *Route of administration*: External application, enema and may be used for *nasya.*
- *Advantage*: It helps in treating *sarvadhatugata vata roga.*

Balaguluchyadi Taila

- *Main ingredients: Bala, guduchi, chandana, ushira* and *yashtimadhu,* etc. processed with milk and oil.
- *Indications:* All *vataja* disorders, *vatarakta* and *raktapitta*
- *Route of administration*: External application and enema
- *Advantage*: Helps in curing *vataja* disorders associated with *pitta* and *rakta.*

Balaswagandha Lakshadi Taila

- *Main ingredients: Ashwagandha, bala, laksha*, etc.
- *Indications:* Insomnia, anxiety neurosis, depression and degenerative disorders like *sandhivata,* in neuromuscular disorders like *pakshaghata* and *ardita,* etc.
- *Route of administration*: External application as well as internally it may be used.
- *Advantage*: It repairs the cartilages. It relieves stress and also reduces pain and inflammation.

Brahmi Taila

- *Main ingredients: Brahmi amalaki,* etc. processed in *tila taila.*
- *Indications:* Stress, insomnia, etc.
- *Route of administration*: External application
- *Advantage*: It is a very good nervine tonic and improves memory, retention power and also induces normal sleep and reduces stress.

Chandanadi Taila

- *Main ingredients: Chandana, madhuka, ashwagandha, koshtha, devadaru*, etc.
- *Indications: Vatarakta, netradaha, angadaha, shirodaha* and *visham jvar*, etc.

- *Route of administration*: External application.
- *Advantage*: It reduces burning sensation and helps in pacification of *rakta* and *pitta*.

Chinchadi Taila

- *Main ingredients: Chincha patra kashaya, shigru, sarjarasa,* etc.
- *Indications:* All *vataja* disorders, especially those associated with *kapha* and *ama*.
- *Route of administration*: External application.
- *Advantage*: Useful in curing *sarvagata, vataja* disorders associated with *kapha* and *ama*.

Dashmula Taila

- *Main ingredients: Dashmula, rasna, eranda,* etc.
- *Indications:* All *vataja* disorders,
- *Route of administration*: External application, enema.
- *Advantage*: Useful in *vataja* disorders associated with degeneration of joints and bones.

Dhanwantara Taila

- *Main ingredients: Bala, kshira and yava, kulatha* and *Baer*, etc.
- *Indications:* All *vataja* disorders, *marma vikara,* in postnatal condition as part of *sutika paricharya,* in neonates, *yoni roga, mutraghata* and psychiatric conditions like *unmada*, etc. It is also useful in *asthi vikara,* where *brihana* is expected.
- *Route of administration*: External application, enema and may be used internally.
- *Advantage*: It can also be used as *avarti kalpana* for internal use.

Dhanwantara Taila (101)

Same as *Dhanwantara taila,* but used internally.

Dhanwantara Kuzhambu

- *Main ingredients: Bala, kshira, yava, kulatha* and *baer*, etc. processed in *yamaka* form.
- *Indications:* Pure *vataja* disorders, degenerative disc diseases, osteo-arthritis and chronic rheumatic conditions

- *Route of administration:* External application only and are preferable to use in *sthanik vasti* procedures.
- *Advantage:* Provides strength to the part, reduces pain

Dhurdhurapatradi Coconut *Taila*

- *Main ingredients: Dhatura patra svarasa* and paste of seeds processed in coconut oil.
- *Indications:* Scaling of scalp, itching of head region.
- *Route of administration*: External application.
- *Advantage*: It is beneficial in psoriatic conditions of scalp and dandruff.

Eladi Taila

- *Main ingredients:* Both types of *ela, kushtha, jatamansi, tagara, guggulu,* etc.
- *Indications:* In *vatakaphaja* disorders, itching, and other skin disorders.
- *Route of administration*: External application.
- *Advantage*: It improves texture and color of skin and increases glow.

Gandha Taila

- *Main ingredients:* Sesame seeds (Tila), cow's milk, *madhuka, nalada, valaka, lohitayashtika, plava, eladi gana, kushta, atibala, mahabala, aguru, durva,* etc.
- *Indications:* All *vataja* disorders, fractures
- *Route of administration*: Internally
- *Advantage*: It is mainly targeted towards improving bone mass and strength. It is useful in the treatment of arthritis, osteoporosis, fractures and dislocations. It is also used in the treatment of ligament injuries.

Himasagara Taila

- *Main ingredients: Shatavari, vidari, kushmanda, dhatri, narikela rasa, lavanga, karpoora,* etc.
- *Indications:* Various neuromuscular conditions and *vata* diseases. It is an excellent pain and burning sensation relieving oil.
- *Route of administration*: Only external application.
- *Advantage*: It is used to treat bone and joint injuries caused by fall, excessive travelling. It is used to treat locomotor problems, chest injury, emaciation, muscle wasting, locked jaw, frozen neck, frozen shoulder, speech difficulties, etc.

Jatamansi Taila

- *Main ingredients: Jatamansi.*
- *Indications:* Stess, anxiety disorders, insomnia, pakshaghata, etc.
- *Route of administration*: External application
- *Advantage*: Gives excellent results when used for *shirodhara* in anxiety, stress and insomnia.

Jatyadi Taila

- *Main ingredients: Jati, nimba, patola, manjishtha*, etc.
- *Indications:* It heals wounds quickly. It is used to apply externally over nonhealing wounds, sinus, blisters, abscess, bite wounds, etc. It is also useful in burns.
- *Route of administration*: External application.
- *Advantage*: It is applied over infected skin diseases such as hand foot and mouth disease, eczema, syphilis, etc. Also beneficial in primary burns.

Jeevanthyadi Yamakam

- *Main ingredients: Taila, ghrita, arka, jivanti, manjista, darvi, kampillaka, tuttha, sarjasara*, etc.
- *Indications:* Cracked feet, hands and lips psoriasis, short sightedness.
- *Route of administration*: External application and *nasya*
- *Advantage*: It is used in various skin ailments, e.g. eczema, psoriasis, contact dermatitis, hives and allergic rashes, etc. also in short sightedness.

Karpasasthyadi Taila

- *Main ingredients: Karpasa bija, bala, masha, kulattha, rasna, koshtha, sarshapa*, etc.
- *Indications:* All *vataja* disorders especially, *avabahuka, pakshaghata* and *ardita*
- *Route of administration*: External application, enema.
- *Advantage*: It is beneficial in neuromuscular disorders like paralysis, frozen shoulder and facial palsy

Karpasasthyadi Kuzhambu

- *Main ingredients: Karpasa bija, bala, masha, kulattha, rasna, koshtha, sarshapa*, etc. processed in *yamaka* form

- *Indications:* All *vataja* disorders especially, *avabahuka, pakshaghata* and *ardita*
- *Route of administration*: External application, enema.
- *Advantage*: It is beneficial in neuromuscular disorders like paralysis, frozen shoulder and facial palsy. It gives better results when used in the cases of muscular weakness/wasting associated with above disorders.

Karpooradi Taila

- *Main ingredients: Kapoor* (Camphor) processed in coconut oil.
- *Indications:* Muscular pain, rheumatoid complaints, joint pain, joint and muscle stiffness.
- *Route of administration*: External application.
- *Advantage*: It is applied to chest to relieve chest congestion. It has got rubefacient effect. Improves blood circulation and brings about warmth. It is used to relieve neck pain, back pain, and multiple joint pains. Excellent for cramps and numbness.

Kottamchukkadi Taila

- *Main ingredients: Kushtha, shunthi, vacha, shigru, lashuna sarshapa* and *rasna*, etc. processed in *dadhi* and *chincha svarasa*.
- *Indications:* All *vataja* disorders, painful conditions associated with inflammatory changes.
- *Route of administration*: External application.
- *Advantage*: It reduces pain and stiffness with great efficacy, also reduces inflammation.

Kshara Taila

- *Main ingredients: Svarjika kshara, romaka lavana, hingu, shigru, devadaru,* etc.
- *Indications:* It is used in ear conditions such as itching, pus, infection, otitis, tinnitus, ear ache, deafness and worms, etc.
- *Route of administration*: External application.
- *Advantage*: Useful for *karnapoorana* in cases of deafness. Good application in facial and dental ailments.

Ksheerabala Taila

- *Main ingredients: Balamula, ksheera, taila*
- *Indications:* All types of *vataja* disorders, osteoarthritis, pakshaghata, ardita, etc.

- *Route of administration*: External application, internally or through enema
- *Advantage*: Beneficial in chronic as well as acute painful rheumatic conditions, paralysis and tetanus, etc. Can be used in Avarti form like ksheerbala 3,7,14,21,101, etc.

Ksheerabala Taila (7/11/101)

Same as that of *ksheerbala taila* but used for orally for internal use.

Kumkumadi Taila

- *Main ingredients: Keshar, chandana, laksha, manjishtha*, etc. processed in *aja* milk and *taila.*
- *Indications:* Hyperpigmentation, dull skin, scars, uneven skin tone.
- *Route of administration*: External application.
- *Advantage*: Improves skin complexion and texture. Relieves blemishes, acne, acne scars, white and black heads, dark circle, sun tans, wrinkles. It has both cleansing and nourishing effect on skin. It has anti-aging qualities

Lakshadi Taila

- *Main ingredients: Laksha, ushira, bala, daruharidra, shatavari,* etc.
- *Indications: Jirnajvara, kshaya, unmada, shvasa, apasmara,* etc
- *Route of administration*: External application
- *Advantage*: It is beneficial in fever and asthmatic conditions.

Mahamasha Taila

- *Main ingredients: Masha, ajamansarasa, dashmula,* etc. processed in cow's milk and *tila taila.*
- *Indications:* All *vataja* disorders like *sandhigata vata, siragatavata, pakshaghata, ardita,* etc.
- *Route of administration*: External application, enema and may be used internally
- *Advantage*: It is excellent *vataghna* oil. It helps in reducing pain and stiffness and also nourishes the tissues. Very good for conditions like varicose veins, paralysis and where muscle wasting is present.

Marichyadi Taila

- *Main ingredients: Marisha, ela, gomutra, sarshapa taila,* etc.

- *Indications:* In various types of skin diseases like *shitapitta* (urticaria), eczema, scabies, etc.
- *Route of administration*: External application
- *Advantage*: Reduces itching immediately after application.

Murivenna Taila

- *Main ingredients: Karanja, tambula, kumari, shigru, kanjika, shatavari,* etc. processed in coconut oil.
- *Indications:* It is a mainly useful in nonhealing wounds, fractures, sprains and blunt injuries.
- *Route of administration*: External application or may be used internally.
- *Advantage*: It is used for application over fresh wounds, old non-healing wounds. It quickens the process of wound healing. It also relieves pain and inflammation in fractures/sprains and promotes healing. It is a very good pain relieving oil.

Nalpamaradi Coconut *Taila*

- *Main ingredients: Triphala, kshirivriksha, kushtha, chandana, manjishtha, ardra haridra,* etc. processed in coconut oil.
- *Indications: Pama, kushtha, pidika, visarpa.*
- *Route of administration*: External application.
- *Advantage*: It has great efficacy in reducing scaling and lesions associated with psoriasis.

Narayana Taila

- *Main ingredients: Aswagandha, bala, bilba, patala, kantakari, gokshura, syonaka, atibala,* etc.
- *Indications:* All types of *vataja* disorders including *yoni roga.*
- *Route of administration*: External application, enema and may be used internally.
- *Advantage*: Enhances cutaneous and capillary blood circulation, adds strength. It strengthens nerves, muscles and ligaments. It relieves muscle and joint stiffness. It reduces pain and inflammation.

Neelibringadi Coconut *Taila*

- *Main ingredients: Neeli, bhringaraja, indralata, amlaki* processed in coconut oil and cow's and buffalo's milk.

- *Indications: Khalitya* and *palitya*.
- *Route of administration*: External application.
- *Advantage*: Helps in reducing hair loss and also delays greying of hair.

Panchavalkala Coconut *Taila*

- *Main ingredients: Panchavalkala, haridra, sariva, kadlikanda, chandana*, etc. processed in coconut oil.
- *Indications: Raktapitta, udara, kushtha, visarpa* with *kleda*.
- *Route of administration*: External application.
- *Advantage*: It is beneficial in curing psoriatic lesions with discharge.

Pinda Taila

- *Main ingredients: Moma* (wax), *sariva, manjistha* and *sarjarasa*, etc.
- *Indications: Vatarakta*, inflammatory conditions of joints.
- *Route of administration*: External application.
- *Advantage*: It contains anti-inflammatory and blood purifying agents so may be used in all conditions of pain associated with inflammation especially in burning pains.

Prabhanjana Vimardhana Taila

- *Main ingredients: Bala, shatavari, shigru, arka, eranda, prasarini, ashwagandha*, etc. processed with *kanji*, cow's milk, *dadhi* and *taila*.
- *Indications: Grivagata vata, vataja vidradhi, vataja gulma, ardita* and pains.
- *Route of administration*: External application
- *Advantage*: It is especially beneficial in diseases related to spine and joints with conditions with muscular stiffness.

Prasarini Taila

- *Main ingredients: Prasarini, meda, mahameda, shatapushpa, rasna*, etc.
- *Indications:* All *vataja* disorders.
- *Route of administration*: External application.
- *Advantage*: It is used to treat locked jaw, stiffness in lower back, sciatica, limping, kyphosis, paraplegia, facial palsy, stiffness in head and neck. It is also useful in treating women infertility, helps in easier conception, and to overcome vaginal ailments. In men, it helps to rectify sperm impurities.

Sahacharadi Kuzhambu

- *Main ingredients: Sahachara, dashmoola, satavari* in *yamaka* form.
- *Indications:* In *vata - kaphaja* disorders, chronic *Ama/srotorodha* conditions and chronic rheumatic pains.
- *Route of administration*: External application, enema therapy
- *Advantage*: It is useful in flaccidity of muscles, esp. rheumatism of lower body and spinal conditions.

Sahacharadi Taila

- *Main ingredients: Sahachara, dashmoola, satavari,* etc.
- *Indications: Kampa, akshepa, stambha, shosha, gulma, unmada, pinasa, yoni roga* and rheumatic pains.
- *Route of administration*: External application, enema and may be used internally.
- *Advantage*: Flaccidity of muscles, rheumatism of lower body. It is also beneficial in conditions associated with *kapha* and *ama.*

Saindhavadi Taila (Brihat)

- *Main ingredients: Saindhava lavana, kanji, mastu* (curd water), rasna, etc. processed with *eranda* (castor) *taila.*
- *Indications:* It is used in the treatment of low back ache, sciatica, rheumatoid arthritis, abdominal colic, ankylosing spondylosis and such other musculoskeletal diseases.
- *Route of administration*: External application, enema and may be used internally.
- *Advantage*: Useful in *vata kaphaja* disorders and conditions associated with *ama.*

Shadbindu Taila

- *Main ingredients: Ajakshira, taila, rasna, bhringaraja, eranda, saindhva,* etc.
- *Indications:* Headache, dizziness, migraine, teeth weakness.
- *Route of administration*: *Nasya* and external application.
- *Advantage*: Helps to cure all types of shirorogas, prevents hair fall, gives strength to the hair roots and teeth, sharpens eyesight. It also gives strength to the shoulders and used in treating avabahuka.

Suddhabala Taila

- *Main ingredients: Balamula* processed in cow's milk and *taila*.
- *Indications:* All *vataja* disorders, *garbhini*, and *prasuta*. Also helpful in treatment of neurological conditions such as hemiplegia, paraplegia, neuralgia, etc.
- *Route of administration*: External application, enema and may be used internally.
- *Advantage*: Beneficial in giving strength to muscles and joints. Also helps uterus to achieve its normal state back after delivery.

Triphaladi Taila

- *Main ingredients: Triphala, guduchi, ketaki, bala eranda, haritaki svarasa*, cow's milk and *taila*.
- *Indications: Shiroroga, pratishyaya, khalitya, palitya* and *medoroga*.
- *Route of administration*: External application, enema.
- *Advantage*: It helps in curing various *urdhvajatrugata roga* and is beneficial in obesity, can be used for *vasti* and massages to achieve weight and inch loss.

Vishagarbha Taila

- *Main ingredients: Dhatura svarasa, kanji, koshtha, bala*, etc processed in *tila taila*.
- *Indications:* Joint pains, stiffness, rheumatic conditions.
- *Route of administration*: External application.
- *Advantage*: It is advised for application on painful conditions of amavata.

GHRITA (MEDICATED GHEE)

Mahatiktaka Ghrita

- *Main ingredients: Saptaparna, ativisha, shampaka, tiktarohini, patha, musta, ushira, triphala, patola, kiratatikta*, etc. processed in *amalaki phala rasa* and *ghrita*.
- *Indications:* It is used as *shamana* and also as *shodhana* medicine in *abhyantara snehakarma* for the treatment of skin diseases, bleeding disorders, bleeding piles, herpes, gastritis, gout, anemia, blisters, schizophrenia, jaundice, fever, heart diseases, menorrhagia. It is highly effective in chronic diseases. It can also be used for application on nonhealing lesions of psoriasis.

Panchatiktak Ghrita

- *Main ingredients: Nimba, patola, vyaghri, guduchi, vasa* processed with *triphala* and *ghrita.*
- *Indications:* It is used for both *shamana* and *shodhana* for treatment of various skin disorders, *pittaja* disorders, worm infestations, hemorrhoids, nonhealing ulcers and cough.

Tiktak Ghrita

- *Main ingredients: Patola, nimba,* katuka, *darvi, duralabha, parpata, trayamana, trayanti, musta, bhunimba, kalinga, kana,* etc. processed in *ghee.*
- *Indications:* It is used for the treatment of skin diseases, *visarpa,* burning sensation, dizziness, itching, anemia, wound with pus, sinus, abscess, blisters, inflammation, psychosis, eye diseases, leucoderma, jaundice, fistula, leucorrhea, piles, etc.

Triphaladi Ghrita

- *Main ingredients: Triphala, bhringaraja swarasa, vasa rasa, shatavari, ajakshira, guduchi rasa, kana, sita, draksha, utpala, madhuka, kshirakakoli,* etc. processed with *ghrita.*
- *Indications:* For treatment of eye diseases and obesity. It can also be used for *akshitarpana* to improve vision.

Jatyadi Ghrita

- *Main ingredients: Jati, nimbapatra, patolapatra, katuka, darvi, nisha, sariva, manjishta, abhaya, siktaka, tuttha, madhuka, naktahva,* etc. processed with *ghrita.*
- *Indications:* It is used externally in the treatment of deep seated wounds and ulcers, nonhealing wound with secretions. It also pacifies pitta.

Jeevanthyadi Ghrita

- *Main ingredients: Jivanti, triphala, daruharidra, pippali,* cow's milk, etc. processed with *ghrita.*
- *Indications:* It is used for the treatment of early stage of cataract. It controls many *pitta*-based ailments. This gives vitality. It can also be used for *akshitarpana* to improve vision.

Shatavaryadi Ghrita

- *Main ingredients: Shatavari, shvadanshtra, vidari, kakoli, ksheerkakoli,* cow's milk, etc. processed with *ghrita.*
- *Indications:* It is useful in treating urinary tract diseases, difficulty in urination, gonorrhea and calculi. Also useful in curing burning sensation of stomach (*amlapitta*) and promotes healthy digestion.

Indukanta Ghrita

- *Main ingredients: Putika, daru, dashamoola,* cow's milk, *pippali, pippalimula, chvya, chitraka, shunthi, yavakshara,* etc. processed in *ghrita.*
- *Indications:* It is useful for treatment of abdominal pain, chronic fever, bloating, weakness and tiredness. It also gives strength to vocal cords. For cough in the aged, this works better than the decoction of the same name. In daily doses, it can cure *jirna javara.*

Kalyanak Ghrita

- *Main ingredients: Triphala, vishala, bhadra ela, devadaru, haridra, sariva, manjishtha,* etc. processed in ghrita.
- *Indications:* It is used for the treatment of cough, anemia, epilepsy, psychiatric disorders, infertility, inflammatory conditions, fever, lack of memory, etc.

Sukumar Ghrita

- *Main ingredients: Punarnava, bilva, patala, shyonaka, agnimantha, gambhari, guda* (jaggery), etc. processed in *ghrita.*
- *Indications:* It is used for the treatment of lower abdominal pain in women, abscess, hemorrhoids, menstrual pain, inflammation, constipation.

OTHER MATERIALS REQUIRED

1. *Dashmula kvath*
2. *Rasnadi kvath*
3. *Manjishthadi kvath*
4. *Kottamchukadi churna*
5. *Kolakulatthadi churna*
6. *Rasnadi churna*

7. *Eladi churna*
8. *Upnaha churna*
9. *Trinapanchamula kvath*
10. *Haltrikadi kvath*
11. *Haridra*
12. *Mthika*
13. *Sarshapa*
14. *Saindhav lavana*
15. *Ajmoda*
16. *Amlaki*
17. *Shatahva*
18. *Balamula*
19. *Ashvagandha mula*
20. *Rasna*
21. *Erandamula*
22. *Nirgundi leaves*
23. *Eranda leaves*
24. *Arka leaves*
25. *Dhattura leaves*
26. *Vacha*
27. *Masha*
28. *Mudga*
29. *Shalishashtika* rice
30. *Godusdha*
31. *Takra*
32. *Musta*

CHAPTER

5 Diet and Regime

According to *Ayurveda*, diet and regime play an important role in the formation of a disease as well as its cure. It is observed that people who give little or no thought towards the diet and regime, they are more prone to make errors unless warned and fall ill.

While undergoing *panchakarma* treatment, it is very important to follow a disciplined routine and diet patterns to allow the body to heal properly and have lasting results. If a person is not careful in following these routines, the results are not satisfying and, at times, can cause aggravation of a disorder.

This is the reason why *deepana* and *pachana* are a must at the beginning of a treatment. As a preparatory measure, a week before the beginning of a *panchakarma* treatment, one should be given medications which felicitate easy and complete evacuation of bowels. It results in cleansing of the intestines and helps in better absorption of "*sara*" (active principles of diet) part of diet into the system.

The following diet and daily regime is mostly advised for all types of *panchakarma* procedures, even though the therapies differ from each other and cater to different types of diseases. They help in achieving the best results if followed properly.

All the restrictions should be followed properly during the treatment and for equal number of days after the treatment is finished to achieve long-lasting results. These restrictions are related not only to diet but also daily regimen and physical and mental activities/exertion.

Lukewarm water or water boiled with *dhanyaka* (coriander), ginger, and cumin seeds should be used for drinking purpose. For washing, bathing and cleaning purposes also only lukewarm water should be used while undergoing these treatments.

Patient should be advised to follow the *ashta mahadoshkar bhava* which are as under:

- Do not speak in loud voice.
- Do not travel by horse, elephant or motorbike, scooter, etc.

- Do not travel or walk in excess.
- Do not sit in one position and on one seat for long hours or duration.
- Do not eat before first meal is already digested.
- Do not eat unhealthy and nonsuitable food.
- Do not sleep in day time.
- Do not engage in coitus.

Patient refrains from suppressing any natural urges such as that urine, hunger; defecation, etc. should be avoided at all the times, physical exertions, mental excitements such as grief, anger, etc. and exposure to cold, dew, sun, wind, smoke or dust should also be avoided.

It was advised to avoid riding on elephants or horses in ancient times, which may relate to distant traveling or traveling short distances in uncomfortable vehicles which may put a person under physical stress should be avoided. It is also advised not to speak aloud or for long durations and any other similar action which may put a system under exertion should also be avoided.

Sleeping during day time and especially after eating food, to stay awake late at night, sitting or standing for long durations or sitting in a wrong posture must also be avoided. One should refrain from using a pillow which is either too high or too low when going to sleep. Any kind of mental exertion or distress should be avoided and the patient must try to be cheerful and happy and wear clean fresh clothes.

WHAT IS THE RIGHT KIND OF FOOD?

It is advisable to take the food which is advised in accordance with *pathya-apathya* of the disease. One should have only such diet as is relishing, yet taking care not to use any article contraindicated by the disease, they should also be easily digestible. Food must be taken in smaller quantities at regular intervals. Food materials that are liquid/semi-solid in form, hot when served, and those that do not cause any *vidaha* should be preferred as far as possible.

While the quality of the food taken is restricted according to the disease, the quantity is also of the utmost importance. One should have food which is wholesome and satisfactory by the moment of eating. Generally, it is advisable, that only half the capacity of the appetite should be filled with solid part of food, one-fourth with liquid and remaining one-fourth should be left empty. This division helps in proper digestion of the food and also results in better absorption of digested material from the intestines. Food materials which are either too spicy/ acidic or fried should always be avoided.

It is important to have a well-balanced diet with the right amount of protein, carbohydrates and fats. Proteins are abundant in peas, beans and other vegetables rich in nitrogen and also in milk, cheese and nuts. However, nuts should be taken according to the season. If accustomed there is no harm in using meat of the *jangala* variety, once a day for patients with strong digestive power. However, it is advisable to take it every second day or twice a week for weaker people. The meat should be broiled, boiled or baked and not fried as, sometimes, it can cause digestive disorders. Veal, pork, fish should be avoided as much as possible as they can cause *raktadushti* as well as indigestion.

Ayurveda strongly advises that milk should never be consumed with meat, fish and salty or sour food articles.

It would be better to avoid all demineralized and fermented foods such as white bread, white crackers and other white flour products. In their place, one should use whole wheat products. Also scoured oatmeal, polished rice, tapioca, yam sweet potato, cornstarch and cornflakes, chillies and tamarind should be avoided and unscoured whole oatmeal, half-polished or brown rice, whole corn meal mush, plantain fruits, black pepper, bitter gourd, snake gourd and other food items containing calcium, magnesium, sodium, iron, potassium, silica and other vital mineral salts should be preferred.

While these cereals and cereal products are protein foods to a considerable extent, they are also carbohydrate and fat foods as they contain various primary food elements in a well-balanced form.

The list of satisfactory health-promoting fats is small, with cream, butter and *ghee* heading the list in digestibility and value. Then there are coconut oil, sesame/mustard and groundnut oil. Animal fats should be used in minimal quantity unless prolonged experience has proven them to be beneficial in a particular case.

Fruits, especially ripe plantain fruits, pomegranates, grapes, oranges and *amalaka* fruits may be eaten, not only for the mineral salts they contain, but also for the stimulating effect, these fruits have upon the liver and other organs of excretion.

While discussing about food, one should also consider the water intake necessary for the proper functioning of digestive and excretory systems. Every person must drink plenty of liquids to help not only digestion but also excretory system. This brings us to another vital point of diet and regime which is discussed below.

USE OF BEVERAGES AND WATER

All stimulants and aerated drinks should be avoided as far as possible. Such things only help to achieve temporary effect and activity and then fall with greater force and reaction.

A frequently asked question in relation to consumption of liquids is whether to drink or not to drink water. It is desirable to drink water while undergoing these treatments to help in detoxification through excretion. It is advisable that if you feel thirst and crave, water, by all the means drink it. But, however, in consideration of the fact that proper diet is to be maintained in order to avoid untoward results, boiled water should be used for drinking purposes. The water for drinking should be boiled with *dhanyaka, sunthi* and *jeeraka* as it also helps in proper digestion of the food.

It is necessary to drink about 10–15 glasses of normal water, preferably between meals everyday for an average person. The best time to drink water is during meals, with possibly one or two glasses during each meal. If drinking of liquids, especially at evening tends to break the sleep by presenting the need to wake up and urinate, it would be advisable to avoid drinking water after dinner, so as to give the kidneys as little to do as possible during the night, though a definite thirst should be satisfied regardless of the time during the day or night.

It would be well to mention here that one of the main reasons for low vitality and lack of resistance is autointoxication from intestinal absorption of waste (toxic) products due to persistent constipated bowels. This condition can be very readily diagnosed, the main symptoms being headache, dizziness, drowsiness, weariness, muscular weakness, nervous irritability, flatulence, foul stools, bad breath, offensive perspiration, irregularities of appetite, furred tongue and disturbed sleep. If any of these symptoms are present in any individual case, it can mostly be noted and absorbed that the patient has constipated bowels.

The predisposing cause of all these troubles is constipation. Constipation arises from over-eating or eating at irregular intervals or the irritability of digestive organs. It leads to lack of ability of the intestines to convert food into easily assimilable and nourishing elements and inability to expel the waste products regularly and in requisite amounts.

However, constipation is one of the systems that tends to develop when these treatments are taken, regardless of the original condition of the bowels. This is mainly due to the restricted diet and exercise.

Under such conditions, it is necessary to have regular and adequate evacuation of the bowels. Even if these symptoms are not present, it is very essential that the bowels be stimulated or rather adjusted to move regularly, during the course of the treatment by the use of a laxative such as "*Gandharvahastadi Kashaya*" so as to ensure satisfactory cleaning of the alimentary tract.

CLOTHING

It is not at all justifiable in swathing oneself in heavy clothing practically blocking air and stop breathing of skin cells. Decently light clothing should be worn, according to the weather. This will allow free entrance of fresh air to the skin cells and facilitate the liberation of the noxious gases thrown off by the skin, the retention of which is as harmful as the swallowing of the same.

By wearing reasonably light cloths the circulation of blood in the skin tissue is improved, the oxidation process of the body is assisted and a more equable degree of warmth is maintained, which is vital for better results of these treatments.

EXERCISE AND RECREATION

One of the foremost essentials of right living is to exercise properly. The main objective of the exercise is to improve the circulation and general nutrition by developing better breathing power and general health.

When undergoing a treatment course, exercises of all forms are strictly forbidden as the body undergoes transitional changes and reconstruction. At that time, the body is in such a condition as it cannot endure the slightest exertion.

Exercise can lead to aggravation of the condition, especially where there is a complete exhaustion of vital forces, or there are neurasthenia and neuralgia to an extreme or muscular condition of heart is dangerously diseased. Also, where movements of the limbs and muscles results in considerable pain, especially of an inflammatory nature, where there is a fever, as in tuberculosis and other acute illnesses and when the blood pressure is high. In these conditions, if strength and general condition permit, some light exercise when taken with proper care and caution can be of some advantage.

If a particular condition necessitates a complete bed rest, it is advisable to take exercise only in the form of passive motion or stretching and tensing of the various muscle groups.

Those who are taking any of these treatments for promotion of health, without having any serious physical disorder, may resort to some sort of light exercises for an hour or so, provided there is no distress during or after the exercise. Also, different types of *yogasanas* may be advised according to the need of a disease wherever possible.

At times, one may feel a "muscular hunger" which passive motion and stretching of the limbs do not fully relieve. In those cases, as well as in any other where it is apparently safe, one may take a short walk in the afternoon, or before retiring, if stirring the sluggish circulation permits. Such light exercise will hasten the progress of the cure by stirring the sluggish circulation and the nerves. Care must be taken, however, to stop the exercise short of the point of actual fatigue, to prevent disturbances and mishaps, which may arise due to exertion.

It is also important to give rest to our sense organs as much as to the body during the course of these treatments to improve their perception capacity.

As food is required as most important part of health so is sleep, the greatest reconstructive factor we have is recovery during sleep, for it is only during sleep that the final processes of assimilation are completed. Six- to-eight hours of sleep at night is necessary for complete rehabilitation of wasted energy and reconstruction and rebuilding of broken down tissues for most people. Sleep in a well-ventilated room, and in a separate bed is always recommended, for the restlessness of one sleeper is likely to affect the other, and the more profound the sleep and least disturbed it is, the quicker and recuperation and the more good one will get out of it.

BATHING

It is advisable not to take a bath immediately after undergoing the treatment. The person undergoing treatment needs to secure more energy to get treated and nourished, which can be achieved by the warm bath taken at a temperature a few degrees above the body heat, or at most, at a temperature not exceeding 110°.

This kind of bath helps in soothing nerves, increases the circulation and promotes free excretion through the pores and causes a general relaxation of all the tissues and organs of the body.

Daily warm water bath is of the most decided advantage in bringing about the best results during the course of the treatment. Especially in almost all conditions characterized with pain and soreness as they promote a better circulation of blood and the pains are eliminated. The bath should be taken only after at least two hours time has lapsed after undergoing the treatment.

It should be realized that when undergoing any of these treatments, one will have little time for other occupations, but if the highest beneficial results are expected, nothing should be allowed to interfere with the treatment. It should be further stressed that social obligation should never interfere with a health restoration program.

Index

Page numbers followed by *f* refer to figure

J

K

L

M

N

O

P

T

U

V